COVID-19 Pandemic
Lessons from the Frontline

T0200459

COVID-19 Pandemic

Lessons from the Frontline

Edited by

Jorge Hidalgo

*General ICU and COVID-19 Unit, Belize Healthcare Partner,
Belize City, Belize*

Gloria Rodríguez-Vega

*Department of Critical Care Medicine, HIMA San Pablo,
Caguas, Puerto Rico*

Javier Pérez-Fernández

*Intensive Care Solutions, Critical Care Services, Baptist
Hospital, Miami, FL, United States*

ELSEVIER

Elsevier
Radarweg 29, PO Box 211, 1000 AE Amsterdam, Netherlands
The Boulevard, Langford Lane, Kidlington, Oxford OX5 1GB, United Kingdom
50 Hampshire Street, 5th Floor, Cambridge, MA 02139, United States

Notices
Knowledge and best practice in this field are constantly changing. As new research and experience broaden
our understanding, changes in research methods, professional practices, or medical treatment may
become necessary.

Practitioners and researchers must always rely on their own experience and knowledge in evaluating and
using any information, methods, compounds, or experiments described herein. In using such information
or methods they should be mindful of their own safety and the safety of others, including parties for whom
they have a professional responsibility.

To the fullest extent of the law, neither the Publisher nor the authors, contributors, or editors, assume any
liability for any injury and/or damage to persons or property as a matter of products liability, negligence or
otherwise, or from any use or operation of any methods, products, instructions, or ideas contained in the
material herein.

Library of Congress Cataloging-in-Publication Data
A catalog record for this book is available from the Library of Congress

British Library Cataloguing-in-Publication Data
A catalogue record for this book is available from the British Library

ISBN: 978-0-323-82860-4

For information on all Elsevier publications visit our
website at https://www.elsevier.com/books-and-journals

Publisher: Dolores Meloni
Acquisitions Editor: Charlotta Kryhl
Editorial Project Manager: Mona Zahir
Production Project Manager: Niranjan Bhaskaran
Cover Designer: Alan Studholme

Typeset by SPi Global, India

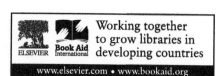

Working together
to grow libraries in
developing countries

www.elsevier.com • www.bookaid.org

We dedicate this book to all frontline workers. Your lessons have shown us that we are all in this together.

Contents

Contributors

Pravin Amin
Bombay Hospital Institute of Medical Sciences, Mumbai, India

Miguel Moreno Aríztegui
Advisor, The President of the Government of Navarra, Pamplona, Spain

Marie R. Baldisseri
Department of Critical care Medicine, University of Pittsburgh Medical Center, Global Health and Disaster Medicine, Pittsburgh, PA, United States

Natalia Largaespada Beer
Ministry of Health, Belmopan, Belize

Erwin Calgua
Research Center of Health Sciences, School of Medicine, University of San Carlos of Guatemala, Guatemala City, Guatemala

María Cruz Martín Delgado
Intensive Care Unit, Hospital Universitario de Torrejón; Universidad Francisco de Vitoria, Madrid, Spain

Fernando Suparregui Dias
Head Critical Care Department, Hospital do Circulo, Caxias do Sul, RS, Brazil

Marilia Díaz
Hospital Auxilio Mutuo; Universidad Sagrado Corazón, San Juan, Puerto Rico

Drew Farmer
Perelman School of Medicine, University of Pennsylvania, Division of Trauma, Surgical Critical Care and Emergency Surgery, Philadelphia, PA, United States

Patxi Pérez Fernández
President, The Association of Journalists of Navarra, Pamplona, Spain

Daniel Godinez
Internal Medicine, Belize Healthcare Partners Limited, Belize City, Belize

Deepa B. Gotur
Department of Medicine, Houston Methodist Hospital, Houston, TX; Weill Cornell Medicine, New York, NY, United States

Sushma Gurav
Ruby Hall Clinic, Pune, Maharastra, India

Erin Hall
Department of Trauma Surgery, Geisinger Medical Center, Danville, PA, United States

John M. Harahus
Geisinger Biocontainment Unit, Geisinger Medical Center, Danville, PA, United States

Allyson Hidalgo
Biochemistry, Arizona State University, Phoenix, AZ, United States

Benjamin Hidalgo
Health Science, Phoenix, AZ, United States

Jorge Hidalgo
General ICU and COVID-19 Unit, Belize Healthcare Partner, Belize City, Belize

Steven H. Hsu
Department of Medicine, Houston Methodist Hospital, Houston, TX; Weill Cornell Medicine, New York, NY, United States

Lewis J. Kaplan
Perelman School of Medicine, University of Pennsylvania, Division of Trauma, Surgical Critical Care and Emergency Surgery, Philadelphia, PA; Society of Critical Care Medicine, Mount Prospect, IL, United States

Ryan J. Logue
Department of Medicine, Houston Methodist Hospital, Houston, TX, United States

Deena Lynch
Brisbane, QLD, Australia

Alexis U. MacDonald
Department Critical Care Medicine, Geisinger Medical Center, Danville, PA, United States

William G. MacDonald
The British East India Company Limited, Birkenhead, Merseyside, United Kingdom

Gerald Marín-García
Critical Care-Emergency Medicine Physician, VA Caribbean Healthcare System, San Juan, Puerto Rico

Ciro Leite Mendes
Head Intensive Care Unit, Hospital Lauro Wanderley, Universidade Federal da Paraíba; Head Intensive Care Unit, Hospital Nossa Senhora das Neves, João Pessoa, PB, Brazil

Andrew Conway Morris
Division of Anaesthesia, Department of Medicine, University of Cambridge; John V Farm Intensive Care Unit, Addenbrooke's Hospital, Cambridge, United Kingdom

Obashina Ogunbiyi
Intensive and Critical Care Society of Nigeria, Benin City, Nigeria

Jose Pascual
Perelman School of Medicine, University of Pennsylvania, Division of Trauma, Surgical Critical Care and Emergency Surgery, Philadelphia, PA, United States

Lorna Pérez
Ministry of Health, Belmopan, Belize

Javier Pérez-Fernández
Intensive Care Solutions, Critical Care Services, Baptist Hospital, Miami, FL, United States

Mary Jane Reed
Geisinger Biocontainment Unit, Geisinger Medical Center, Danville, PA, United States

Gloria Rodríguez-Vega
Department of Critical Care Medicine, HIMA San Pablo, Caguas, Puerto Rico

Regis Goulart Rosa
Intensive Care Unit and Research Projects Office, Hospital Moinhos de Vento, Porto Alegre, RS, Brazil

Michael Singh
Office of the Prime Minister of Belize, Belmopan, Belize

Jacqueline Y. Steuer
Manager Critical Care Services APN team; NorthShore University HealthSystem, Evanston, IL, United States

Rishi Suresh
Texas A&M School of Medicine, College Station, TX, United States

Ahmed Reda Taha
Cleveland Clinic Lerner College of Medicine, Case Western Reserve University, Critical Care Institute, Cleveland Clinic Abu Dhabi, Abu Dhabi, United Arab Emirates

Allison Tong
Sydney School of Public Health, The University of Sydney, Sydney, NSW, Australia

Laila Woc-Colburn
Division of Infectious Diseases, Emory University School of Medicine, Atlanta, GA, United States

Edwin Wu
Intensive Care Solutions, Baptist Hospital, Miami, FL, United States

Kapil Zirpe
Ruby Hall Clinic, Pune, Maharastra, India

Jose Pascual
Perelman School of Medicine, University of Pennsylvania, Division of Trauma, Surgical Critical Care and Emergency Surgery, Philadelphia, PA, United States

Leroe Pérez
Ministry of Health, Belmopan, Belize

Javier Perez-Fernandez
Intensive Care Solutions, Critical Care Services, Baptist Hospital, Miami, FL, United States

Mary Jane Reed
Geisinger Bioconstankship Unit, Geisinger Medical Center, Danville, PA, United States

Elena Rodriguez-Vega
Department of Critical Care Medicine, MMA, San Pedro, Spain; Miami, FL

Rajiv Bhushan Asaa
[affiliation illegible]
Troy, Meyer, NY, United States

Michael Singh
College of the Physic, Medicine, and York, Design San, United

Jacqueline Y. Stoner
Manager Division Care Services ANP, team North Lake, Advent Health, Peoria, IL, United States

Rishi Suresh
[affiliation illegible]

Ahmad Raza Taha
Cleveland Clinic, Lerner College of Medicine, Case Western Reserve University, Critical Care Institute, Cleveland Clinic, Abu Dhabi, Abu Dhabi, United Arab Emirates

Allison Tour
Sydney School of Public Health, The University of Sidney, Surgery, NSW, Australia

Laila Woc-Colburn
Division of Infectious Diseases, Emory University School of Medicine, Atlanta, GA, United States

Erwin Wu
Intensive Care Solutions, Baptist Hospital, Miami, FL, United States

Kapil Zirpe
Ruby Hall Clinic, Pune, Maharashtra, India

Preface

By the end of 2019, the world witnessed the appearance of a new strain of virus causing respiratory and systemic illness in the region of Wuhan, China. Progressively, media attention grew to that area and news were being watched with concern by some and skepticism by others. However, it was not until the latest February and the beginning of March 2020, when the infection spread to Europe and the United States, that the world started to focus attention to this disease. Even then, the media and public opinion were divided into the needs or appropriateness of the responses that different countries were developing about the convenience of border closures or the implementation of quarantine for travelers or even close contacts.

The year of 2020 has been one that humanity will recall as a "dark one," not only by the COVID-19 pandemic but also by the erratic, disorganized, and sometimes misdirected response of public authorities, media, and private individuals. A conglomerate of opinions, the lack of evidence to formulate health-care policies and responses, and the feeling of the absence of international cooperation have been the markers of this year. These represent a motive to learn and evolve for future events to come.

Lessons from the Front Line explores some first-hand experiences, from those who have been involved in this fight, in the first line of the response, from those who have suffered the disease, and from those who have been affected directly or indirectly by the COVID-19 and whose lives have abruptly changed. With the experiences and opinions reflected on the book, we would like to make a call for attention to some aspects that need serious improvement to cope with future disasters, hopefully not to be seen soon.

We have explored the impact of the pandemic into the economy with the political ramifications that have been involved in some policies invoked in the name of health but questionable in their motives and implementations. We have also reflected the experience from those who have worked front line, their opinions, their sorrows, and their suggestions on how to improve our health-care system locally, regionally, and beyond borders. We echoed the thoughts of those who have suffered the disease and rendered their inside feelings into these pages. We have conveyed the voice of media professionals, concerned about the erratic and sometimes misleading information appearing everywhere with a special mention to social media that has revealed an incredible value for true and fake news. Finally, we have incorporated the voice of the professional societies and administrations in an attempt to consolidate and organize future efforts.

We believe that the *Lessons from the Front Line* is a window display of the journey that the world has engaged in 2020, a year that brought up challenges, confusion, deception, and the greatest spirit of mankind. We, the editors, believe that humanity has learnt from our mistakes and that the year 2020 has made us stronger, and we see in all these processes a glimmer of hope for our human race. Together we fight, together we win.

Javier Pérez-Fernández, MD
Jorge Hidalgo, MD
Gloria Rodríguez-Vega, MD

Acknowledgments

Special thanks to the different authors for taking the time to prepare these chapters; despite hectic schedules and busy lives, the completion of this undertaking could not have been possible without your valuable contribution. We want to recognize the great contribution of Pilar Ramón Pardo and PAHO Washington.

We want to offer a special thanks to the guidance provided by Elsevier Staff, especially to Mona Zahir, the editorial project manager, for your patience and your dedication to this project has been helpful, and we feel fortunate to have had the opportunity to work to such a professional group.

Thanks to our families for their unconditional support and encouragement. It is not easy to express our gratitude for all your incredible patience and understanding. They are a constant reminder of what is truly important in life.

The sudden appearance of SARS-CoV-2

Jorge Hidalgo[a], Gloria Rodríguez-Vega[b], and Javier Pérez-Fernández[c]

[a]*General ICU and COVID-19 Unit, Belize Healthcare Partner, Belize City, Belize,* [b]*Department of Critical Care Medicine, HIMA San Pablo, Caguas, Puerto Rico,* [c]*Intensive Care Solutions, Critical Care Services, Baptist Hospital, Miami, FL, United States*

Introduction

Numerous viral infections have risen in the last decades, causing severe diseases associated with lethality. Diseases have varied in epidemiology and morbidity although people with risk factors such as age, cardiovascular diseases, diabetes, and other chronic diseases have most commonly suffered more serious consequences. The world population is aging and so is the prevalence of noncommunicable diseases. Thus, the potential group of people, who are the most at risk of suffering major consequences if infected by a virus, is vast. One such example is the novel coronavirus (nCoV), identified in Wuhan, China, which was isolated on January 7, 2020, causing severe pneumonia.[1]

This chapter analyzes the emergence, first outbreaks outside China, and the epidemiology data and models that has guided public health policies. The period covered in this chapter had included the first notification of cases by China until the declaration of a pandemic by the World Health Organization (WHO) on February 11, 2020. This chapter also describes some of the similarities between this virus and previous coronaviruses (CoVs) like severe acute respiratory syndrome (SARS)-CoV (2002) and middle east respiratory syndrome (MERS)-CoV (2012).

The ancestors: Coronavirus and humans

CoVs, a large family of single-stranded RNA viruses, have been circulating on Earth for centuries. While CoVs are widely detected in bats, other mammals, birds, and reptiles, CoVs are seldom seen in humans causing mainly mild respiratory infections. It was not until the first decade of the twenty-first century with the appearance of the SARS outbreak that their clinical importance was recognized.

Coronaviruses have the largest known RNA genome, with a size of 27–32 kb. The spike glycoprotein (S) protrudes from the surface of the viral particle (hence the name "coronavirus") and is responsible for receptor binding and membrane fusion. Therefore, it is believed to represent a key determinant of host range restriction.[2]

There are four main subgroups of CoVs, namely alpha, beta, gamma, and delta. Human CoVs were first identified in the mid-1960s. Common human CoVs are endemic globally and causing mild respiratory disease are 229E (alpha CoV), NL63 (alpha CoV), OC43 (beta CoV), and HKU1 (beta CoV. They tend to be transmitted predominantly during the winter season in temperate climate countries; they are well adapted to humans, and none have been found to be maintained in an animal reservoir.[3, 4]

On the contrary, SARS-CoV and MERS-CoV are mostly based on zoonotic reservoirs, with occasional spillover into the susceptible human population, possibly via an intermediate host species. Thus, in the first years of this century, SARS-CoV demonstrated that animal CoVs have the potential to cross over species to humans. In the late 2003, angiotensin-converting enzyme 2 was identified as the receptor of SARS-CoV on the surface of human cells, allowing thespillover into humans.[5]

The index cases of many of these SARS-CoV early case clusters (from November 2002 to January 2003) were food handlers working in restaurants where a variety of exotic animals were slaughtered on the premises.[6] In February 2003, the Chinese Ministry of Health announced the strange outbreak of an atypical pneumonia in the Guangdong Province of southern China. News of this "mysterious" disease spread fast, as did the disease. During subsequent weeks, the outbreak became self-sustaining, with clusters of transmission in hospitals spilling back into the community. The identification of the SARS-CoV did not happen until almost three months later (April 2003).[7]

SARS spreads rapidly along routes of air travel, affecting 25 countries and territories across five continents, with an estimated 8096 cases and at least 774 deaths (case fatality rate $\sim 10\%$). The outbreak continued until July 2003, when the WHO declared "all known chains of human-to-human transmission of the SARS virus now appear to be broken."[8] SARS was less transmittable in the first days of illness, leading patients to be more infectious as they became more symptomatic, providing an opportunity for case detection and isolation to interrupt transmission. However, the higher transmission by severe patients has contributed to transmission in hospitals, especially when they underwent aerosol-generating procedures. The SARS-CoV was also unusually lasting on surfaces, more so than other CoVs or other respiratory viruses, making infection control in hospitals a challenge.[9] As awareness grew, patients began to be identified and hospitalized earlier in the illness, and as effective infection control, modalities were better implemented, it became possible to interrupt transmission in the community and hospitals.[10]

The zoonotic source of the virus was identified after the outbreak ended; the investigations led to the detection of the virus in a range of mammalian species available in the wet markets. People working in these markets had a high prevalence of antibodies to SARS-CoV, even without a history of having SARS. SARS-CoV crossed the species barrier into masked palm civets and other animals in live-animal markets in China; genetic analysis suggested that this occurred in the late 2002. Several people in close proximity to palm civets became infected with SARS-CoV.[11]

The emergence of SARS in 2003 demonstrated the interconnection of the world and how rapidly a new disease can spread, due to the exponential increase in international travel and trade. That impulsed the need to review international mechanisms for monitoring and control of emerging diseases; not only for the four serious infectious diseases included in the original International Health Regulations (IHR) from 1969.[12] In 2005, the World Health Assembly, representing 196 countries, agreed to implement the revised IHR as a commitment to build their capacities to detect, assess, and report public health events under a broader range of public health emergency of international concern (PHEIC). The WHO plays the coordinating role in IHR and, together with technical partners, helps countries to build their capacities to detect and contain public health hazards.

Almost a decade later of the SARS-CoV, a new CoV emerged in Saudi Arabia in 2012, subsequently named MERS-CoV. MERS-CoV is a beta-coronavirus, like the SARS-CoV. It causes severe pneumonia as well as renal failure. Index cases have originated in the Arab Peninsula (Jordan, Qatar, Saudi Arabia, and the United Arab Emirates), while travel-associated cases have been diagnosed in the European Union, North Africa, Asia, and the USA. The receptor for MERS-CoV has been identified to be dipeptidyl peptidase IV, which is expressed in the human respiratory tract and is conserved across many species, including bats.[12] This virus, originated from bats, uses camels and dromedaries as intermediary hosts; and, although the outbreak declined over the time, the risk of new cases is still considered to exist as the animal reservoir persists.[13] By the end of December 2019, 27 countries reported a total of 2502 laboratory-confirmed cases of MERS, including 861 associated deaths (case–fatality rate: 34.4%); the majority of these cases were reported from Saudi Arabia (2106 cases, including 783 related deaths, case–fatality rate: 37.2%). Reported cases are classified as primary (direct spillover from camels) or secondary (human-to-human transmission, mostly healthcare workers); the proportion between those categories changed over the time, in the period July–December 2019, 33% were primary cases, 6% were secondary cases, and 31% of unknown contact history. As in SARS-CoV, human-to-human transmission of MERS-CoV occurs mainly associated with healthcare.[14] The predominance of nosocomial transmission is probably due to the fact that higher virus shedding (high viral loads in respiratory tracts) occurs after the onset of symptoms when most patients are already seeking medical care.[15] As an example, in the period 2013–2019, approximately 20% of the cases of MERS were healthcare workers in Saudi Arabia.[16]

Affected countries reduced the global threat of MERS by addressing knowledge gaps about transmission, enhancing surveillance, and strengthening the ability to detect cases early and contain outbreaks through improved infection prevention and control measures in hospitals. Preventing international spread and sustained transmission has been improved by local policies, better prevention and control measures in hospitals, restriction of camel movement in affected areas, stronger and more comprehensive investigations of cases and clusters, and improved communication.[17]

Unfortunately, neither the SARS nor the MERS outbreaks yield to solid clinical data on the efficacy of treatment regimens. This evidence was urgently needed for the treatment of MERS, as well as to prepare for nCoVs that may emerge, as it was demonstrated with SARS-CoV-2.

While MERS has not caused the international panic seen with SARS, the emergence of this second, highly pathogenic zoonotic human CoV illustrates the threat posed by this viral family. In 2017, the WHO placed SARS-CoV and MERS-CoV on its Priority Pathogen list, to accelerate research and the development of vaccines and antivirals against CoVs.[18]

Emergence of SARS-2 CoV

On December 31, 2019, a cluster of cases of pneumonia of unknown etiology–a surveillance definition after the SARS outbreak–were detected in Wuhan City, Hubei Province of China. Patients exhibited symptoms of viral pneumonia including fever, difficulty breathing, and bilateral lung infiltration in the most severe cases. Bronchoalveolar samples from these patients were positive for pan-Beta coronavirus (real-time PCR assays).[19] As of January 20, 2020, 282 confirmed cases of this nCoV have been reported from four countries including China, Thailand, Japan, and the Republic of Korea.[20]

The novel virus was named as Wuhan CoV or 2019 nCoV (2019-nCov) by the Chinese researchers. The International Committee on Taxonomy of Viruses Coronaviridae Study Group has studied the classification of the new virus and named it as "SARS-CoV-2."[21] The disease name (which in many cases is different from the virus name) has been designated as coronavirus disease 2019 (COVID-19) by the WHO. The "19" in COVID-19 stands for the year (2019) that the virus was first seen. The virus name was announced by the WHO on February 11, 2020.[22]

The critical factor for an emergent virus is its pandemic potential. Efficient human-to-human transmission is a requirement for a large-scale spread. The proportion of patients with mild symptoms is another important factor that determines the ability to identify infected individuals and to prevent the transmission of the virus. Identification of transmission chains and subsequent contact tracing are further complicated when several individuals remain asymptomatic or mildly symptomatic.[23]

Genetic studies: Looking for the origin

In less than a month, the nCoV was identified, isolated, and sequenced by the Chinese scientists. The complete viral genome sequences from the initial patients showed a sequence identity of 99.98%.[24] This level of viral genomic identity isolated from different human subjects is unusual for an RNA virus that has been circulating for a long time in the human population. This observation suggests a recent single spillover event from an animal source into humans.

Genetic sequencing of the Wuhan coronavirus offers clues to its origins and spread. With regards to its origin, the alignment of the full-length genome sequence of the SARS-CoV-2 and other available genomes of Beta CoV showed the closest relationship was with the bat SARS-like CoV strain BatCov RaTG13 (identity match 96%) and suggest multiple outbreak sources of transmission.[25]

Nine months after the detection of SARS-CoV-2, laboratories all over the world have sequenced the genomes of more than 5000 strains and have made them publicly available.[26] This phylogeny (Fig. 1) shows evolutionary relationships of SARS-CoV-2 viruses from the ongoing nCoV COVID-19 pandemic; and an initial emergence in Wuhan, China, in November–December 2019 followed by sustained human-to-human transmission leading to sampled infections. Although the genetic relationships among sampled viruses are quite clear, there is uncertainty surrounding estimates of specific transmission dates and in reconstruction of geographic spread.

Viral sequences could identify any genetic changes that might have helped the virus make the jump from animals to humans, and signs that the virus has gained further mutations that are enabling it to spread more efficiently in humans. For instance, the transmission rate of SARS-CoV-2 is higher than SARS-CoV, and the reason could be genetic recombination event at S protein of SARS-CoV-2. The single N501T mutation in SARS-CoV-2's Spike protein may have significantly enhanced its binding affinity for the human angiotensin-converting enzyme 2 protein.[27]

Primary reservoirs and hosts of SARS-CoV-2: A market full of wildlife

The source of the SARS-CoV-2 is still unknown, although the initial cases have been associated with the Huanan Seafood Wholesale Market, Wuhan, China. The live animals are frequently sold at the Huanan Seafood Wholesale Market such as bats, frogs, snakes, birds, marmots, and rabbits.[28] Environmental samples taken from this market in December 2019 tested positive for SARS-CoV-2, further suggesting that the market in Wuhan City was the source of this outbreak or played a role in the initial amplification of the outbreak, but no specific animal association has been identified.[29–31]

Genetic sequencing suggests that the SARS-CoV-2 is related to CoVs that circulate in bats, including SARS and its close relatives. Probably, the lineage giving rise to SARS-CoV-2 has been circulated unnoticed in bats for more than 40 years. SARS-CoV-2 itself is not a recombinant of any sarbecoviruses (the viral subgenus containing SARS-CoV and SARS-CoV-2) detected to date, and its receptor-binding motif, important for specificity to human angiotensin-converting enzyme 2 receptors, appears to be an ancestral trait shared with bat viruses and not one acquired recently via recombination.[32]

Besides bats, other mammals can transmit these viruses and, similarly to SARS, SARS-CoV was most likely to spread to humans by mammals. Claims were made but were not substantiated that snakes or pangolins[33] were intermediate hosts for

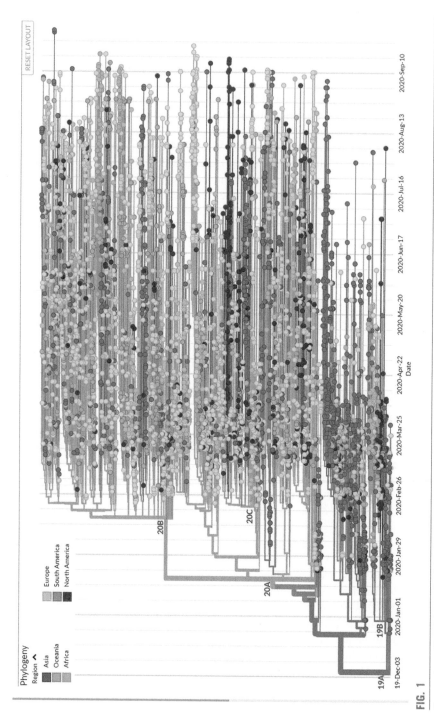

FIG. 1

Genomic epidemiology of nCoV. Phylogenic tree as of September 2020.

Credit: https:/nextstrain.org/ncov/global.

creating the coronavirus by recombination events.[34] Researchers are currently working to identify the source of 2019-nCoV including possible intermediate animal vectors.

In addition to investigations on the possible intermediate host(s) of SARS-CoV-2, there are also a number of studies underway to better understand the susceptibility of SARS-CoV-2 in different animal species. Current evidence suggests that humans infected with SARS-CoV-2 can infect other mammals, including dogs, cats, ferrets, and farmed mink.[35–38]35 However, it remains unclear if these infected mammals pose a significant risk for transmission to humans.

The source of origination and mechanisms of zoonotic transmission are important to be determined in order to develop preventive strategies to contain the infection; from prevention of additional zoonotic exposures/risk exposure, infection prevention and control measures, nonpharmacological measures, and the development of vaccines in adequate animal models.

Human-to-human transmission

Initially, most of the early COVID-19 patients in China had an epidemiological link with the Wuhan market: they may have visited the wet market where live animals were sold or may have used infected animals or birds as a source of food. However, none of the exported cases had contact with the market, and early epidemiological studies showed that there was an exponential increase in the number of cases beginning in the late December 2019 clearly suggesting the human-to-human spreading capability of this virus since the middle of that month.[39, 40] To identify the transmission mechanism is extremely relevant for the implications in infection prevention precautions and to determine the specific measures and efforts to reduce transmission would be required to control outbreaks.

The transmission mechanism among humans was early identified as respiratory. The human-to-human spreading of the virus occurs in close contact with an infected person, exposed to coughing, sneezing, respiratory droplets, or aerosols. These particles can penetrate the human body via inhalation through the nose or mouth initiating their replication in the mucosa cells of the respiratory tract.[41, 42] Contact transmission (direct contact with an infected subject or indirect contact, through hand-mediated transfer of the virus from contaminated fomites to the mouth, nose, or eyes) is considered very likely, given consistent findings on environmental contamination in the vicinity of infected cases and the fact that other coronaviruses and respiratory viruses can transmit this way. However, there are no specific reports that have directly demonstrated fomite transmission. People who touch potentially infectious surfaces often have close contact with the infectious person, making the distinction between respiratory droplet and fomite transmission difficult to discern. Lastly, indirect transmission through fomites is considered possible, although, so far, transmission through fomites has not been documented.[36]

Infection is understood to be mainly vectored via large respiratory droplets containing the SARS-CoV-2 virus. Transmission through aerosols (droplet nuclei that remain infectious when suspended in air over long distances and time) can occur during medical procedures that generate aerosols. WHO, together with the scientific community, has been actively discussing and evaluating whether SARS-CoV-2 may also spread through aerosols in the absence of aerosol generating procedures, particularly in indoor settings with poor ventilation. There is no evidence of aerosol transmission in the absence of aerosol generating procedures.[43]

As SARS-CoV-2 has been found in the fecal samples, the possibility of fecal–oral (including waterborne) transmission needs to be considered. A scoping review showed that the virus is less stable in the environment and is very sensitive to oxidants, like chlorine, and temperature (the titer of infectious virus declines more rapidly at $23\,°C–25\,°C$ than at $4\,°C$).[44] There is no current evidence that human coronaviruses are present in surface or groundwater bodies or are transmitted through contaminated drinking water.

Virus transmissibility and RO estimations

Early epidemiological records in China suggest that up to 85% of human-to-human transmission occurred in family clusters. Healthcare workers became infected with an absence of major nosocomial outbreaks and some supporting evidence that some healthcare workers acquired infection in their families.[37] These findings suggest that close and unprotected exposure is required for transmission by direct contact in the immediate environment of those with infections.

Continuing reports from outside China suggest the same means of transmission to close contacts and persons who attended the same social events or were in circumscribed areas such as office spaces or cruise ships.[38, 45] Therefore, it looks like that transmission rates are higher in closed settings than in open air ones.

Transmissibility is measured by two parameters: secondary attack rate and basic reproduction number (R0). Attack rate has been measured in different settings, such as attendees of a religious event (estimated attack rate 38%–78%) or children attending summer camp (estimated attack rate 44%).[46, 47] SARS-CoV-2 spread efficiently in both settings, resulting in high attack rates among persons in all age groups. Asymptomatic infection was common and potentially contributed to undetected transmission.

R0 is considered as one of the most valuable parameters to predict the evolution of an epidemic, useful to answer questions about how fast the disease will spread or estimating other response parameters such as the number of hospital beds needed. Its value has important implications for predicting and measuring the effects of pharmaceutical and nonpharmaceutical interventions. R0 has been extremely difficult to estimate at the beginning of the pandemic because of the underreporting of asymptomatic and mild cases. This parameter is often calculated as a fixed property of a pathogen, based on the mode of transmission; but R0 also depends on the behavior (i.e., how often people come into contact with one another) that can differ drastically between countries, cities, or neighborhoods. For instance, the European Center for Disease Prevention and Control and other researchers, initially estimated the R0 for COVID-19 to be between 2 and 3 as per the epidemiological data from China.[48, 49]

However, soon other studies estimated R0 using multiple methods and reported large-scale outbreak with R0 equal to 6.47 [95% confidence interval (CI) 5.71–7.23] or 5.7 (95% CI 3.8–8.9) indicating higher transmission of COVID-19. That highlights the importance of active surveillance, contact tracing, quarantine, and early strong social distancing efforts to stop transmission of the virus.[50, 51]

Controversies about transmission
People without symptoms

Once the human-to-human mechanism transmission was clear, another major discussion over transmission was whether—and how extensively—people without symptoms can infect others.[39] Infected persons without symptoms could play a significant role in the ongoing pandemic, but their relative number and effect have been under discussion. As early as February 2020, it was evidence that people infected with SARS-CoV-2 who did not develop symptoms of COVID-19, but whose viral load was similar to that of symptomatic cases, suggesting a potential for transmission.[52, 53] If such asymptomatic cases are common and these individuals can spread the virus, then containing its spread will be much more difficult. In that context, the proportion of asymptomatic persons who tested positive for SARS-CoV-2 infections was estimated to account for approximately 40%–45%, and they can transmit the virus to others for an extended period, perhaps longer than 14 days.[40] These are people fully asymptomatic, not the ones who will develop symptoms later on (presymptomatic). Research has shown that people become infectious before they start feeling sick, during that presymptomatic period. The difficulty of distinguishing asymptomatic persons from those who are merely presymptomatic is extremely an obstacle in epidemiological or clinical studies, leading to acknowledge the possibility that some of the proportions of asymptomatic persons are lower than reported, as those who are presymptomatic cases.

Children and transmission

Currently, the extent to which children contribute to transmission of SARS-CoV-2 overall remains unclear. The contribution of children at the total of cases and deaths is minimal (1.7% of cases and less than 1% of the deaths).[54–56] On the other hand, evidence is limited regarding the prevalence of SARS-CoV-2 infections in children, but it appears to be lower for younger children (e.g., under 12 years old) compared to the adult population (above 18 years old) and teenagers (13–19 years old).[41–43] Despite the high viral load detected in children, their contribution to transmission is not clear, as the evidence suggests that most cases in children result from household exposures, and transmission among children and staff in educational settings is low.[55]

Contact tracing provides an accurate estimate on transmission. In South Korea, tracing of 59,073 contacts of 5706 index patients detected COVID-19 in 11.8% of household contacts. In children, the highest COVID-19 rate (18.6% [95% CI 14.0%–24.0%]) was found for household contacts of school-aged children (10–19) and the lowest (5.3% [95% CI 1.3%–13.7%]) for household contacts of children aged 0–9 years in the middle of school closure. These data suggest that children younger than 10 years transmit the virus to others in the household much less often than adults do, but the risk is not zero.[44]

Transmission is influenced by many other factors as well, such as droplet production, physical environment (air flow, temperature, and humidity), susceptibility of the exposed person, transmission greatly influenced by activities, and social behavior patterns. In summary, the degree to which age alone, regardless of symptoms, affects viral load, and thus, the infectiousness of COVID-19 remains unclear.

In conclusion, although the rise in cases probably reflects an increase in testing, the dramatic jump seen in many countries is concerning. The researchers are struggling to accurately model the outbreak, and to predict how it might unfold, because the case report data are incomplete (date of starting of symptoms and proportion of asymptomatic cases).

Early dissemination—The first outbreaks

Once human-to-human transmission was documented by the first epidemiological studies, it was clear that the transmissibility of the virus was high. In its early stages, the epidemic doubled in size for every 7.4 days.[57] In this section, it describes the local and international COVID-19 dissemination until the declaration of pandemic by WHO (March 11, 2020).

China

About the dynamics of the transmission in China, the WHO Joint Mission (February 16–242,020) informed on the transition from early cases identified in Wuhan are believed to have acquired the infection from a zoonotic source, as many reported visiting or working in the Huanan Seafood Wholesale Market.[51] However, early in the outbreak, the cases generated human-to-human transmission chains that seeded the subsequent community outbreak. The dynamics of transmission radiated from Wuhan to other parts of Hubei province and China. On January 23, 2020, Wuhan city was locked down—with all travel in and out of Wuhan prohibited—and movement inside the city was restricted with the purpose of preventing further transmission. Within Hubei, the implementation of control measures (including social distancing) reduced the community force of infection, resulting in the progressively lower incident reported case counts.

Given Wuhan's transport hub status and population movement during the Chinese New Year, infected individuals quickly spread throughout the country and were particularly concentrated in cities with the highest volume of traffic with Wuhan.[51]

Based on the epidemiological official data, the published literature, and on-site visits in Wuhan (Hubei), Guangdong (Shenzhen and Guangzhou), Sichuan (Chengdu), and Beijing, the Joint WHO China Mission team made the following epidemiological observations on the demographic characteristics of the 55,924 laboratory-confirmed cases reported as of February 20, 2020. The median age was 51 years (range from 2 days to 100 years old; interquartile range 39–63 years old) with the majority of cases (77.8%) aged between 30 and 69 years. Among the reported cases, 51.1% were male, 77.0% were from Hubei, and 21.6% were farmers or laborers by occupation.

The data are similar to the first series of cases published by the Chinese Center for Disease Control and Prevention.[58] By February 11, 2020, a total of 72,314 individuals diagnosed with COVID-19 were included in the analysis. Among them, 44,672 cases (61.8%) were confirmed, 16,186 cases (22.4%) were suspected, 10,567 cases (14.6%) were clinically diagnosed, and 889 cases (1.2%) were asymptomatic. Most of the confirmed cases ($N = 44{,}672$) were aged 30–69 years (77.8%), male (51.4%), farmers or laborers (22.0%), and diagnosed in the Hubei Province (74.7%). Most patients reported Wuhan-related exposures (85.8%) and were classified as mild cases (80.9%). The lethality rate was estimated to be around 2.3% (confirmed cases). Of all the age groups, the patients in the $\geq$80 years age group had the highest case fatality rate at 14.8%. The case fatality rate for males was 2.8%, and for females, it was 1.7%. While patients who reported no comorbid conditions had a case fatality rate of 0.9%, patients with comorbid conditions had much higher rates—10.5% for those with cardiovascular disease, 7.3% for diabetes, 6.3% for chronic respiratory disease, 6.0% for hypertension, and 5.6% for cancer.

In the first WHO Situation Report on the nCoV, dated January 20, 2020, there were reports of confirmed cases from three countries outside China: Thailand, Japan, and South Korea.[59] These cases had all been exported from China, with no documented local transmission outside China yet.

On January 30, 2020, the WHO has declared this first outbreak of nCoV in China a PHEIC.[46] This is a formal declaration of "an extraordinary event which is determined to constitute a public health risk to other states through the international spread of disease and to potentially require a coordinated international response," formulated when a situation arises that is "serious, sudden, unusual, or unexpected," which "carries implications for public health beyond the affected state's national border" and "may require immediate international action."[47] Under the 2005 IHR, states have a legal duty to respond promptly to a PHEIC. As this is a new coronavirus, the global community should demonstrate solidarity and cooperation, in compliance with Article 44 of the IHR (2005), in supporting each other on the identification of the source of this new virus, its full potential for human-to-human transmission, preparedness for potential importation of cases, and research for developing necessary treatment. Under Article 43 of the IHR, States Parties implementing additional health measures that significantly interfere with international traffic (refusal of entry or departure of international travelers, baggage, cargo, containers, conveyances, goods, and the like, or their delay, for more than 24 h) are obliged to send to WHO the public health rationale and justification within 48 h of their implementation.

During the following weeks, several countries implemented entry screening measures for arriving passengers from China. Soon, several major airlines suspended their flights from and to China.[48]

Travel restrictions were issued to impede or slow down transmission in a number of countries. As mentioned, on January 23, 2020, Wuhan City was locked down—with all travel in and out of Wuhan prohibited—and movement inside the city was restricted. The major problem for airport control would be that about 64% of the infected travelers were presymptomatic at arrival, as estimated per Monte Carlo simulation.[49] Therefore, travel restrictions are insufficient to contain the global spread of COVID-19, as it was later on demonstrated. With most cases arriving during the asymptomatic incubation period, rapid contact tracing would be essential both within the epicenter and at importation sites to limit human-to-human transmission outside of mainland China. Modeling suggested that sustained 90% travel restrictions modestly affect the epidemic trajectory unless combined with a 50% or higher reduction of transmission in the community.[50]

In less than 8 weeks, the overall number of cases reported as of March 10, 2020 was 113,702 confirmed cases with 4012 deaths. Of those, in China, there were 80,924 confirmed cases with 3140 deaths, while outside of China 32,778 confirmed cases with 872 deaths. About 109 countries/territories/areas have reported the confirmed cases of COVID-19. The most affected countries after China were the Republic of Korea (7513), Iran (7161), and Italy (9172) (Figs. 2 and 3). The WHO risk assessment at national, regional, and global level was very high.

Asia

After the announcement of 41 confirmed COVID-19 cases in Wuhan City, China on January 11, infected patients were identified in Thailand on January 8 and 13.[51] According to the cases' history, the two imported COVID-19 cases described were not directly linked, yet their genomes were identical. They had no direct link to the Huanan Seafood Wholesale Market, but their genomes were identical to four sequences from Wuhan collected on December 30, 2019, indicating potential wider distribution in the city.

The first imported case of COVID-19 in Japan was reported on January 3, with laboratory confirmation on January 16th, and notified the WHO.[59] The patient did not visit the seafood market. However, he potentially had close contact with pneumonia patients during his stay in Wuhan, raising the possibility of human-to-human spread. Both Thailand and Japan are among the top three Wuhan air travel destinations, according to a study on travel patterns and public health preparedness in light of the new threat.

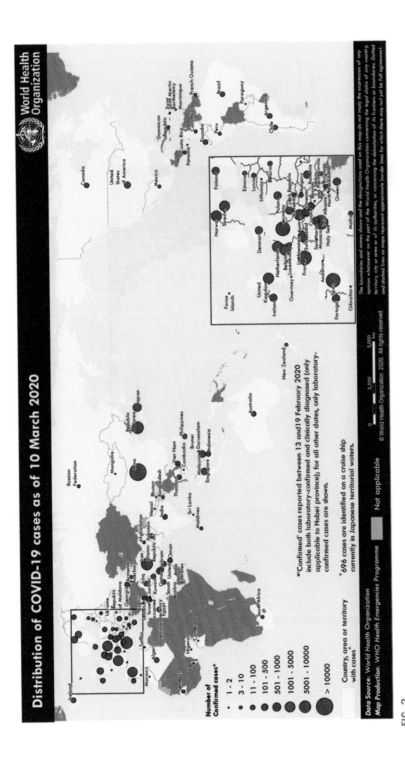

Distribution of COVID-19 cases as of 10 March 2020

World Health Organization

Number of Confirmed cases*

- · 1 - 2
- · 3 - 10
- ● 11 - 100
- ● 101 - 500
- ● 501 - 1000
- ● 1001 - 5000
- ● 5001 - 10000
- ● > 10000

● Country, area or territory with cases*

Data Source: World Health Organization
Map Production: WHO Health Emergencies Programme

Not applicable

*"Confirmed" cases reported between 13 and 19 February 2020 include both laboratory-confirmed and clinically diagnosed (only applicable to Hubei province); for all other dates, only laboratory-confirmed cases are shown.

+ 696 cases are identified on a cruise ship currently in Japanese territorial waters.

0   2,500   5,000
                    km

© World Health Organization 2020. All rights reserved.

The boundaries and names shown and the designations used on this map do not imply the expression of any opinion whatsoever on the part of the World Health Organization concerning the legal status of any country, territory, city or area or of its authorities, or concerning the delimitation of its frontiers or boundaries. Dotted and dashed lines on maps represent approximate border lines for which there may not yet be full agreement.

FIG. 2

Countries, territories with reported confirmed COVID-19 cases as of March 10, 2020.

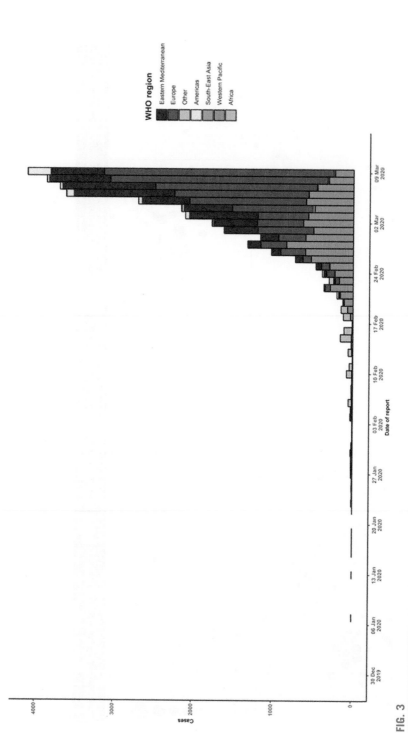

FIG. 3

Epidemic curve of confirmed COVID-19 cases ($N = 32,778$) reported outside of China, by date of report and WHO region with complete days of reporting through March 10, 2020.

Credit: WHO.

In Korea, 28 confirmed cases of COVID-19 had been reported as of February 14, since the first case was confirmed on January 20, 2020. Of these, 16 cases were imported into the country (57.1%) and 10 were believed to be secondary cases of infections originating in Korea; in the other 2 cases, the route of transmission remained undetermined.[60] At that point, these COVID-19 cases originating in Korea have been reported to be index cases imported from abroad, and resultant first-generation and second-generation cases.

Europe

The first infections in Europe occurred between January 16 and 24 by a group of 30 tourists from Wuhan visiting Italy, Switzerland, and France. The first European case was reported in France on January 24, 2020. This case had a travel history to China. In Germany, cases were reported on January 28, related to a person visiting from China.

In the WHO European Region, COVID-19 surveillance was implemented on January 27, 2020. As of February 21, nine European countries reported 47 cases. Among 38 cases studied, 21 were linked to two clusters in Germany and France, 14 were infected in China.[64] The median age of the case was 42 years; 25 were male. Late detection of the clusters' index cases delayed isolation of further local cases. As of March 5, there were 4250 cases. The analysis of early cases, we observed transmission in two broad contexts: sporadic cases among travelers from China (14 cases) and cases who acquired infection due to subsequent local transmission in Europe (21 cases).[64]

As of March 2, the European Center for Diseases Prevention and Control reported about the increasing number of countries with widespread community transmission around the world and in Europe, and these are exporting cases with subsequent transmission to previously unaffected areas. Only 9 days later, as of March 11, all the European countries were affected, reporting a total of 17,413 cases and 711 fatalities. Italy represented 58% of the cases ($N = 10,149$) and 88% of the fatalities ($N = 631$).[52]

Iran

Iran reported its first two CoV cases on February 19, 2020. The virus may have been brought to the country by a traveler to China. Less than a week later, the country reported to WHO 61 COVID-19 cases and 12 related deaths. Iran borders are crossed each year by millions of religious pilgrims, migrant workers, and others. As of March 1, 2020, Iran had reported 987 novel (COVID-19) cases, including 54 associated deaths. At least six neighboring countries (Bahrain, Iraq, Kuwait, Oman, Afghanistan, and Pakistan) had reported imported COVID-19 cases from Iran. Researchers and modelers used air travel data and the numbers of cases from Iran imported into other Middle Eastern countries to estimate the number of COVID-19 cases.[53]

The national authorities reported an increasing number of new cases and deaths, reaching 8042 cases and 291 deaths on March 11.[61]

America

https://www.cdc.gov/mmwr/volumes/69/wr/mm6918e2.htm.

https://www.contagionlive.com/news/most-early-new-york-covid-19-cases-came-from-europe.

USA early transmission

Latin America

Caribbean

In light of this situation, Pan American Health Organization's Alert in January 16, 2020 recommended the Member States to strengthen surveillance activities to detect any unusual respiratory health event.[65] Health professionals should be informed about the possibility of the occurrence of infection caused by this virus and the actions to be implemented in case of a suspected case.

Transmission in cruises

Cruise ships are often settings for outbreaks of infectious diseases. The spread of SARS-CoV-2 in cruise ships, in particular in the Diamond Princess, provided very rich information on the transmission and characterization of the clinical spectrum, in particular of the asymptomatic cases. On February 5, 2020, in Yokohama, Japan, a cruise ship hosting 3711 people underwent a 2-week quarantine after a former passenger was found with COVID-19 post-disembarking. At the end of the quarantine, 634 persons on board tested positive for SARS-CoV-2. It was estimated that each infected passenger infected 11 others. On March 10, 7 deaths caused by the virus were registered. The estimated asymptomatic proportion was 17.9% (95% CI15.5%–20.2%).[54]

During the initial stages of the COVID-19 pandemic, the Diamond Princess was the setting of the largest outbreak outside mainland China. Many other cruise ships have since been implicated in the SARS-CoV-2 transmission, such as the Grand Princess cruise ship. As of March 17, confirmed cases of COVID-19 had been associated with at least 25 additional cruise ship voyages. More than 800 cases and 10 deaths of laboratory-confirmed COVID-19 cases occurred during outbreaks on these cruise ship voyages until the end of March 2020.[55]

From outbreak(s) to pandemic

Since the WHO declared this first outbreak of nCoV a "PHEIC" on January 30, there were increasing reports globally informing on the local transmission in multiple locations, without reported travel history to areas reporting community transmission and without epidemiological links to known cases. Several countries implemented entry screening measures for arriving passengers from China, and soon, several major airlines suspended their flights from and to China, although these public health measures did not prevent the dissemination of the virus across the globe. Events and locations that involve social interaction or institutional contact have been related to the development of COVID-19 clusters, including workplace interactions, religious events, festivities, health and social care settings, and travel. Transmission events were reported in hospitals, with COVID-19 cases identified among healthcare workers and patients as well as in long-term care facilities.[56] Considering the global spread with the local transmission, the Director General of the WHO declared COVID-19 as a global pandemic on March 11, 2020.[62]

The spread of the virus was exponential. Despite of the Chinese government efforts meeting the international standards in terms of isolation of suspect cases, diagnosis and treatment and educational campaigns, only 2 months after the notification of the first COVID cases through IHR, as of March 1, 2020, the local transmission was reported in 13 countries outside of China such as South Korea, Japan, Singapore, Australia, Malaysia, Vietnam, Italy, Germany, France, the United Kingdom, Croatia, San Marino, Iran, the United Arab Emirates, and the United States of America.[63] The most worrisome evidence was the local transmission documented in multiple locations and extensively, without direct or indirect epidemiological link to China. Only 10 days later, as of March 11 more than 118,000 cases of COVID-19 were reported worldwide in 114 countries, with 4291 fatalities.[63,64] By then, it was clear that the world was entering a new phase of the global outbreak. Efforts to restrict the COVID-19 virus to China had failed, and in some countries, the focus had to turn towards mitigation rather than containment, as they try to slow the spread of the infection to stop hospitals all being overwhelmed at once. At that point, the WHO made the declaration of pandemic. Nevertheless, describing the situation as a pandemic did not change WHO's assessment of the threat posed by this virus, nor did the WHO recommendations and technical support to the countries change.

This expanding epidemic has been a stress test for existing health systems, including those of industrialized countries. It has also provided further motivation to strengthen fundamental research in trans-species viral infections and on potential zoonosis impacts, particularly from bats, under changing environmental conditions.

Acknowledgments

Special Thanks: Dr. Pilar Pardo and PAHO Washington for the enormous contribution to make this chapter possible.

References

1. World Health Organization. *Novel Coronavirus (2019-nCoV). Situation report-1. 21 January*; 2020. [cited 2020 June 29] Available from: https://www.who.int/docs/default-source/coronaviruse/situation-reports/20200121-sitrep-1-2019-ncov.pdf?sfvrsn=20a99c10_4.
2. Hilgenfeld R, Peiris M. From SARS to MERS: 10 years of research on highly pathogenic human coronaviruses. *Antiviral Res.* 2013;100(1):286–295. https://doi.org/10.1016/j.

antiviral.2013.08.015. ISSN 0166–3542, [cited 2020 July 1] Available from: https://www.sciencedirect.com/science/article/pii/S0166354213002234.

3. Shuo S, Wong G, Shi W, et al. *Epidemiology, Genetic Recombination, and Pathogenesis of Coronaviruses, Trends in Microbiology*. Vol. 24; 2016:490–502. Issue 6. ISSN 0966-842X. [cited 2020 1 July] Available from https://www.sciencedirect.com/science/article/pii/S0966842X16000718.

4. de Wit E, van Doremalen N, Falzarano D, Munster VJ. SARS and MERS: recent insights into emerging coronaviruses. *Nat Rev Microbiol*. 2016;14(8):523–534. https://doi.org/10.1038/nrmicro.2016.81.

5. Li W, Moore MJ, Vasilieva N, et al. Angiotensin-converting enzyme 2 is a functional receptor for the SARS coronavirus. *Nature*. 2003;426:450–454.

6. Xu RH, He JF, Evans MR, et al. Epidemiologic clues to SARS origin in China. *Emerg Infect Dis*. 2004;10:1030–1037.

7. Peiris JS, Lai ST, Poon LL, et al. Coronavirus as a possible cause of severe acute respiratory syndrome. *Lancet*. 2003;361:1319–1325.

8. https://www.who.int/features/2003/07/en/.

9. Cheng PK, Wong DA, Tong LK, et al. Viral shedding patterns of coronavirus in patients with probable severe acute respiratory syndrome. *Lancet*. 2004;363:1699–1700.

10. Leung GM, Hedley AJ, Ho LM, et al. The epidemiology of severe acute respiratory syndrome in the 2003 Hong Kong epidemic: an analysis of all 1755 patients. *Ann Int Med*. 2004;141:662–673.

11. Hilgenfeld R, Peiris M. From SARS to MERS: 10 years of research on highly pathogenic human coronaviruses. *Antiviral Res*. 2013;100(1):286–295. ISSN 0166-3542 https://doi.org/10.1016/j.antiviral.2013.08.015. [cited 2020 July 1] Available from: https://www.sciencedirect.com/science/article/pii/S0166354213002234.

12. Wang N, Shi X, Jiang L, et al. Structure of MERS-CoV spike receptor-binding domain complexed with human receptor DPP4. *Cell Res*. 2013;23:986–993.

13. Killerby ME, Biggs HM, Midgley CM, et al. Middle East respiratory syndrome coronavirus transmission. *Emerg Infect Dis*. 2020;26(2):191–198. https://doi.org/10.3201/eid2602.190697.

14. Yin Y, Wunderink RG. MERS, SARS and other coronaviruses as causes of pneumonia. *Respirology*. 2018;23(2):130–137. https://doi.org/10.1111/resp.13196.

15. de Wit E, van Doremalen N, Falzarano D, Munster VJ. SARS and MERS: recent insights into emerging coronaviruses. *Nat Rev Microbiol*. 2016;14(8):523–534. https://doi.org/10.1038/nrmicro.2016.81.

16. World Health Organization. *Regional Office for the Eastern Mediterranean, MERS situation update*; 2019. [cited 2020 30 June]. Available at: https://applications.emro.who.int/docs/EMCSR246E.pdf?ua=1&ua=1.

17. Donnelly CA, Malik MR, Elkholy A, et al. Worldwide reduction in MERS cases and deaths since 2016. *Emerg Infect Dis*. 2019;25(9):1758–1760. https://doi.org/10.3201/eid2509.190143.

18. World Health Organization. *Annual review of disease prioritized under the Research and Development Blueprint. Informa consultation. 6-7 February 2018*; 2018. Geneva, Switzerland. [cited 2020 1 July] Available from: http://origin.who.int/emergencies/diseases/2018prioritization-report.pdf.

19. Tan W, Zhao X, Ma X, et al. A novel coronavirus genome identified in a cluster of pneumonia cases—Wuhan, China 2019–2020. *China CDC Weekly*. 2020;2(4):61–62. https://doi.org/10.46234/ccdcw2020.017.

20. World Health Organization. *Novel Coronavirus (2019-nCoV). Situation Report - 1*; 2020. 21 January. [cited 2020 July 1] Available from: https://www.who.int/docs/default-source/coronaviruse/situation-reports/20200121-sitrep-1-2019-ncov.pdf?sfvrsn=20a99c10_4.

21. Gorbalenya AE, Baker SC, Baric RS, et al. The species *Severe acute respiratory syndrome-related coronavirus*: classifying 2019-nCoV and naming it SARS-CoV-2. *Nat Microbiol.* 2020;5:536–544. https://doi.org/10.1038/s41564-020-0695-z.

22. World Health Organization. *Novel Coronavirus (2019-nCoV) Situation Report - 22*; 2020. 11 February [cited 2020 July 1] Available from: https://www.who.int/docs/default-source/coronaviruse/situation-reports/20200211-sitrep-22-ncov.pdf?sfvrsn=fb6d49b1_2.

23. Munster VJ, Koopmans M, van Doremalen N, van Riel D, de Wit E. A novel coronavirus emerging in China—key questions for impact assessment. *N Engl J Med.* 2020;382 (8):692–694.

24. Lu R, Yu X, Wang W, et al. Characterization of human coronavirus etiology in Chinese adults with acute upper respiratory tract infection by real-time RT-PCR assays. *PLoS ONE.* 2012;7(6). https://doi.org/10.1371/journal.pone.0038638, e38638.

25. Kim JS, Jang JH, Kim JM, Chung YS, Yoo CK, Han MG. Genome-wide identification and characterization of point mutations in the SARS-CoV-2 genome. *Osong Public Health Res Perspect.* 2020;11(3):101–111. https://doi.org/10.24171/j.phrp.2020.11.3.05.

26. https://nextstrain.org/ncov/global.

27. Wan Y, Shang J, Graham R, Baric RS, Li F. Receptor recognition by novel coronavirus from Wuhan: an analysis based on decade-long structural studies of SARS. *J Virol.* 2020.

28. Gralinski LE, Menachery VD. Return of the coronavirus: 2019-nCoV. *Viruses.* 2020;12 (2):135. https://doi.org/10.3390/v12020135.

29. World Health Organization. *Novel Coronavirus (2019-nCoV) Situation Report - 94*; 2020. 23 April [cited 2020 July 1] Available from: https://www.who.int/docs/default-source/coronaviruse/situation-reports/20200423-sitrep-94-covid-19.pdf?sfvrsn=b8304bf0_4.

30. Andersen KG, Rambaut A, Lipkin WI, Holmes EC, Garry RF. The proximal origin of SARS-CoV-2. *Nat Med.* 2020;26(4):450–452.

31. Zhou P, Yang X-L, Wang X-G, et al. A pneumonia outbreak associated with a new coronavirus of probable bat origin. *Nature.* 2020;579(7798):270–273.

32. Boni MF, Lemey P, Jiang X, et al. Evolutionary origins of the SARS-CoV-2 sarbecovirus lineage responsible for the COVID-19 pandemic. *Nat Microbiol.* 2020. https://doi.org/10.1038/s41564-020-0771-4.

33. Zhang T, Wu Q, Zhang Z. Probable pangolin origin of SARS-CoV-2 associated with the COVID-19 outbreak. *Curr Biol.* 2020;30:1346–1351. e2.

34. Brüssow H. The novel coronavirus—a snapshot of current knowledge. *Microb Biotechnol.* 2020;13(3):607–612. https://doi.org/10.1111/1751-7915.13557.

35. Oreshkova N, Molenaar R-J, Vreman S, et al. SARS-CoV2 infection in farmed mink, Netherlands, April 2020 (pre-print). *BioRxiv.* 2020. https://doi.org/10.1101/2020.05.18.101493.

36. World Health Organization. *Transmission of SARS-CoV-2: implications for infection prevention precautions. Scientific Brief. 9 July*; 2020. Available in: https://www.who.int/publications/i/item/modes-of-transmission-of-virus-causing-covid-19-implications-for-ipc-precaution-recommendations.

37. Zhang J, Litvinova M, Wang W, et al. Evolving epidemiology and transmission dynamics of coronavirus disease 2019 outside Hubei province, China: a descriptive and modelling study. *Lancet Infect Dis.* 2020;S1473–3099(20):30230–30239. [Epub ahead of print]. doi:10.1016/S1473-3099(20)30230-9.

38. Rothe, Schunk M, Sothmann P, et al. Transmission of 2019-nCoV infection from an asymptomatic contact in Germany. *N Engl J Med.* 2020;382:970–971.

39. The National Institute of Infectious Diseases Japan. Field briefing: Diamond Princess COVID-19 cases. n.d. https://www.niid.go.jp/niid/en/2019-ncov-e/9407-covid-dp-fe-01.html.

40. Callaway E, Cyranoski D. China coronavirus: six questions scientists are asking. *Nature.* 2020. 22 January. Update 28 January 2020. [cited 2020 1 July] Available from: https://www.nature.com/articles/d41586-020-00166-6#ref-CR4.

41. Oran DP, Topol EJ. Prevalence of asymptomatic SARS-CoV-2 infection: a narrative review. *Ann Intern Med.* 2020. https://doi.org/10.7326/M20-3012. 32491919.

42. Stringhini S, Wisniak A, Piumatti G, et al. Seroprevalence of anti-SARS-CoV-2 IgG antibodies in Geneva, Switzerland (SEROCoV-POP): a population-based study. *Lancet.* 2020;396(10247):313–319.

43. Public Health England. *Weekly Coronavirus Disease 2019 (COVID-19) Surveillance Report. Summary of COVID-19 surveillance systems*; 2020.

44. Pollán M, Pérez-Gómez B, Pastor-Barriuso R. Prevalence of SARS-CoV-2 in Spain (ENE-COVID): a nationwide, population-based seroepidemiological study. *Lancet.* 2020. https://doi.org/10.1016/S0140-6736(20)31483-5.

45. Park YJ, Choe YJ, Park O, et al. Contact tracing during coronavirus disease outbreak, South Korea, 2020. *Emerg Infect Dis.* 2020. https://doi.org/10.3201/eid2610.201315. Oct [date cited].

46. Li Q, Guan X, Wu P, et al. Early transmission dynamics in Wuhan, China, of novel coronavirus-infected pneumonia. *N Engl J Med.* 2020;382(13):1199–1207. https://doi.org/10.1056/NEJMoa2001316.

47. The Novel Coronavirus Pneumonia Emergency Response Epidemiology Team. The epidemiological characteristics of an outbreak of 2019 novel coronavirus diseases (COVID-19)—China, 2020. *China CDC Weekly.* 2020;2(8):113–122. https://doi.org/10.46234/ccdcw2020.032.

48. World Health Organization. *COVID -19 Situation Report # 1*; 2020. 21 January. Available from: https://www.who.int/docs/default-source/coronaviruse/situation-reports/20200121-sitrep-1-2019-ncov.pdf?sfvrsn=20a99c10_4.

49. World Health Organization. *COVID -19 Situation Report # 11*; 2020. 31 January. Available from https://www.who.int/docs/default-source/coronaviruse/situation-reports/20200131-sitrep-11-ncov.pdf?sfvrsn=de7c0f7_4.

50. World Health Organization n.d. https://www.who.int/ihr/procedures/pheic/en/.

51. Phelan AL, Katz R, Gostin LO. The novel coronavirus originating in Wuhan, China: challenges for global health governance. *JAMA.* 2020.

52. Wells CR, Sah P, Moghadas SM, et al. Impact of international travel and border control measures on the global spread of the novel 2019 coronavirus outbreak. *Proc Natl Acad Sci.* 2020;117(13):7504–7509. https://doi.org/10.1073/pnas.2002616117.

53. Chinazzi M, Davis JT, Ajelli M, et al. The effect of travel restrictions on the spread of the 2019 novel coronavirus (COVID-19) outbreak. *Science.* 2020;368(6489):395–400. https://doi.org/10.1126/science.aba9757. https://science.sciencemag.org/content/368/6489/395.

54. Pilailuk O, Rome B, Siripaporn P, et al. Early transmission patterns of coronavirus disease 2019 (COVID-19) in travelers from Wuhan to Thailand, January 2020. *Euro Surveill.* 2020;25(8):2000097. https://doi.org/10.2807/1560-7917.ES.2020.25.8.2000097.

55. COVID-19 National Emergency Response Center, Epidemiology and Case Management Team, Korea Centers for Disease Control and Prevention, Korea Centers for Disease Control and Prevention, Cheongju, Korea. *Osong Public Health Res Perspect.* 2020;11(1):8–14. https://doi.org/10.24171/j.phrp.2020.11.1.03.

56. European Centre for Disease Prevention and Control. *Novel coronavirus disease 2019 (COVID-19) pandemic: increased transmission in the EU/EEA and the UK – sixth update – 12 March 2020.* Stockholm: ECDC; 2020.

57. Zhuang Z, Zhao S, Lin Q, et al. Preliminary estimation of the novel coronavirus disease (COVID19) cases in Iran: a modelling analysis based on overseas cases and air travel data. *Int J Infect Dis.* 2020;94:29–31.

58. World Health Organization. *COVID -19 Situation Report # 51*; 2020. 11 March. Available from: https://www.who.int/docs/default-source/coronaviruse/situation-reports/20200311-sitrep-51-covid-19.pdf.

59. Kenji M, Katsushi K, Alexander Z, Gerardo C. Estimating the asymptomatic proportion of coronavirus disease 2019 (COVID-19) cases on board the Diamond Princess cruise ship, Yokohama, Japan, 2020. *Euro Surveill.* 2020;25(10):2000180. https://doi.org/10.2807/1560-7917.ES.2020.25.10.2000180.

60. Moriarty LF, Plucinski MM, Marston BJ, et al. Public health responses to COVID-19 outbreaks on cruise ships—worldwide, February–March 2020. *MMWR Morb Mortal Wkly Rep.* 2020;69:347–352. https://doi.org/10.15585/mmwr.mm6912e3.

61. European Centre for Disease Prevention and Control (ECDC). *Outbreak of novel coronavirus disease 2019 (COVID-19): increased transmission globally – fifth update.* Stockholm: ECDC; 2020. 2 March. Available from: https://www.ecdc.europa.eu/sites/default/files/documents/RRA-outbreak-novel-coronavirus-disease-2019-increase-transmission-globally-COVID-19.pdf.

62. WHO Director-General's opening remarks at the media briefing on COVID-19 - 11 March; 2020. https://www.who.int/dg/speeches/detail/who-director-general-s-opening-remarks-at-the-media-briefing-on-covid-19- - -11-march-2020.

63. World Health Organization (WHO). *Coronavirus disease 2019 (COVID-19) - Situation Report - 40*; 2020. Available from: https://www.who.int/docs/default-source/coronaviruse/situationreports/20200229-sitrep-40-covid-19.pdf?sfvrsn=7203e653_2.

64. European Centre for Disease Prevention and Control (ECDC). *Outbreak of novel coronavirus disease 2019 (COVID-19): increased transmission globally – fifth update.* Stockholm: ECDC; 2020. 2 March. Available from: https://www.ecdc.europa.eu/sites/default/files/documents/RRA-outbreak-novel-coronavirus-disease-2019-increase-transmission-globally-COVID-19.pdf.

65. A pandemic in all but name. *New Scientist.* 2020;245(3271):5. Available online 28 February https://doi.org/10.1016/S0262-4079(20)30423-1. https://www.sciencedirect.com/science/article/pii/S0262407920304231?via%3Dihub.

COVID-19 disaster preparedness

Alexis U. MacDonald[a], John M. Harahus[b], Erin Hall[c], Mary Jane Reed[b], and Marie R. Baldisseri[d]

[a]*Department Critical Care Medicine, Geisinger Medical Center, Danville, PA, United States,*
[b]*Geisinger Biocontainment Unit, Geisinger Medical Center, Danville, PA, United States,*
[c]*Department of Trauma Surgery, Geisinger Medical Center, Danville, PA, United States,*
[d]*Department of Critical care Medicine, University of Pittsburgh Medical Center, Global Health and Disaster Medicine, Pittsburgh, PA, United States*

Disaster has been defined in numerous terms. But in essence, disaster is a disruption of function that causes the ability of the affected community to overcome using its resources.[1] Pandemics are considered progressive occurrences with one causal organism, but various reasons for expanding from local infectious outbreak to a global pandemic. Unlike natural disasters, which most often have definitive onset and known number of immediately affected populations, epidemics most often begin sporadically and increase based on the route of transmission, infectivity, and mitigation efforts. This variability can complicate all stages of the disaster cycle (Fig. 1).

All disaster preparedness begins with basic concepts. Chance of the hazard or event happening to an area and the vulnerability of that community in the event of that event. This is termed the hazard vulnerability analysis (HVA). Novel infectious outbreaks such as coronavirus disease 2019 (COVID-19) are difficult because transmission, at-risk population, natural history, and effective public health policies are unclear early in the course. This leads to short or even nonexistent time to do an HVA. Before COVID-19, the 2019 U.S. National Health Security Preparedness Index, which assesses the ability to provide health care during large-scale public health threats, reported a significant gap in the U.S. health-care system to maintain quality health care during and after such an event.[2] This chapter gives the authors' perspective of how our systems approach disaster planning to the COVID-19 pandemic. Both health systems have multiple hospitals that overlap in Pennsylvania, which experienced a surge of COVID-19 patients early in the United States. The University of Pittsburgh Medical Center (UPMC) is urban based, while Geisinger Medical Center is rural based. Both systems' hospitals and their communities are historically interconnected.

Proper preparation, resource allocation, and education contribute to variability and disaster response. Several studies from natural disasters show that resiliency and collaboration can support recovery efforts for communities. Some communities face unique challenges such as rural locations with geographic variability, funding,

COVID-19 Pandemic. https://doi.org/10.1016/B978-0-323-82860-4.00007-0

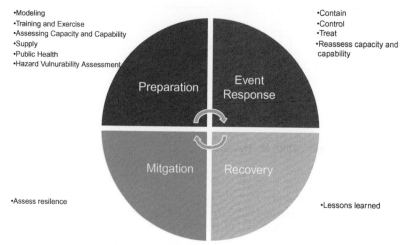

•Modeling
•Training and Exercise
•Assessing Capacity and Capability
•Supply
•Public Health
•Hazard Vulnurability Assessment

•Contain
•Control
•Treat
•Reassess capacity and capability

Preparation

Event Response

Mitgation

Recovery

•Assess resilence

•Lessons learned

FIG. 1

Disaster cycle.

coordination, and cooperation among local networks. The capacity and capability of a community and health system to respond to emergencies determine preparedness. Capacity is defined as having enough personnel and supplies, while capability has the correct resources. Appropriate and timely resource allocation and mobilization are essential steps to ensure preparedness. Unlike natural disasters, epidemics can be prolonged and put extreme pressure on the health systems making mitigation or "flattening the curve" paramount to maintaining capacity and capability.

From prior disaster research and recent COVID-19 experience, several themes emerge. There is extensive variability across the national, local, and organizational levels in addressing preparedness policies. Despite this variability, there is a clear need for essential aspects of preparedness, including assessing resources (stuff/space), training for providers (staff), and increased communication/collaboration across networks/programs. The inadequate response, failure to triage, and lapses in communication are common systemic barriers to significant incidents.[3]

The initial assessment must also include the identification of all stakeholders. The stakeholders include the community, the health-care system, and the local/state/national networks. Each stakeholder group has systemic and organizational structures established to aid in disaster response. In the community, this includes federal, state, and local governments and the community residents.

Community

The community requires information and education about their role in preparation and response. Public health networks and the existing health-care system strive to work in concert to orchestrate disaster response. The success of a coordinated response and action plan is dependent on the strength and stability of the existing networks. Information and education are essential for the community to participate in their protection. Infection control and public health initiatives need to be accurate and timely communicated. Dissemination of precise information must include national and local health-care efforts to support public health. Additional measures by local government and primary care providers can help the community.

Geisinger has a robust connection with the community, given the population that it serves. Through social media and other public forums, Geisinger engages the community. Their participation through public health initiatives, such as universal mitigation strategies, and following local visiting policies are essential to combat surge. Geisinger leadership held community town halls throughout the pandemic to engage the public. Additional challenges to community preparedness are the dissemination of accurate and timely information. During an election year, the political climate can affect the tenor and quality of information that reaches the community. Public health initiatives should strike a neutral tone and be rooted in evidence and science. In the end, the public depends on its health-care system and the institution's preparations.

Health care
Stuff

Health-care preparedness is the analysis and preparation of what is required and anticipated opportunities to plan. Disaster planning includes mobilization of necessary resources. The effective systemic response must have a coordinated and collaborative model to expect future surge. The importance of recognizing the current state versus the predicted future state is essential. Pandemic preparation at our institutions was a multipronged approach. The capability of our existing network to flex and respond requires the understanding of the supply chain and the available resources.

Resources and the delivery of care to patients demand accuracy. Supplies such as equipment, oxygen, and medications must be available as an alternative solution. The disruption of the supply chain during a disaster period also needs to be anticipated. Each department assessed current supplies and leadership focused on policies and procedures to implement throughout the network. For example, our existing triage policy was reviewed and updated by a multidisciplinary team of critical care leadership, physicians, and medical ethicists. Past analysis of disaster preparedness helps inform and prioritize activities that maximize a hospital's capability to respond.[4]

Health-care delivery and estimates for surge capacity are required. Models exist to assist officials both nationally and locally for surge planning tools (PACER). Strategies to improve capacity such as (1) opening unlicensed beds, (2) canceling elective admissions, and (3) implementing reverse triage were all used simultaneously in preparation for the pandemic surge.[5] At the network level, daily communication and collaboration supported our response to meet current needs for intensive care unit (ICU) level of care.

Staff

In the Society of Critical Care Medicine's ICU Readiness Report to evaluate the state of ICU preparedness during the height of the COVID-19 pandemic in March 2020, 82% of respondents reported ICU shortages and bed capacity and 58% reported issues with adequate ICU staffing.[6] Proactive planning for ICU staffing augmentation is paramount to the successful response to a local surge in ICU and critical care patient volumes. Each hospital system must design a system which caters to their personnel needs in terms of physicians, advanced practice providers (APPs), and nursing staff, among others. There will be an array of capabilities based on preexisting personnel, but plans should incorporate contingency plans to add additional personnel who are either present in the hospital working in different roles or with the use of outside personnel via ICU telemedicine. Institutions must have a framework to plan for increased capacity with the proportional expansion of staff and stuff. A framework was recently published, suggesting a tiered/graded system provides adequate staffing structure to respond.[7] The local surge planning involves unit closures and redeployment of employees.

UPMC is a 40-hospital system ranging from rural to tertiary/quaternary academic centers in Pennsylvania, New York, and Western Maryland. They designed and rolled out a system-level ICU pandemic surge staffing algorithmic plan for implementation when "normal" ICU resources were exhausted and the potential for 100%–200% surge increase in patient volume occurs (reference). The plan was developed to ensure that local needs were balanced with system resource supply. A tiered-provider strategy was used by the hospitals to allow for adequate ICU and critical care coverage by physicians and nurses who had some experience in managing acutely ill patients. The first step in designing any staffing plan is to ascertain what were the existing staffing and then determine how this could be augmented with additional providers including tele-ICU medicine capabilities. UPMC used a tiered staffing algorithm designating "Tier 1" providers as critical care providers including telemedicine critical care providers. "Tier 2" providers were identified as those physicians with prior/remote critical care training, experience and skills, other airway capable providers (e.g., certified registered nurse anesthetists), and those who were non-airway providers but were ICU-capable providers (e.g., APPs). A "flex" tier, if available, could be a separate procedure team specifically for intubations, bronchoscopies, central and arterial lines, prone positioning, etc. This flex team could free up procedural time for those critical providers in the ICU and on the ward to focus on clinical management. In Fig. 2, the tiered staffing strategy shows how critical care including mechanical ventilator management be administered to four groups of 24 patients with a team managed by a critical care-trained physician. In Fig. 3, a more detailed outline is presented for the progression from Tier 1 to Tier 3 providers with the possible additional of tele-ICU support as well as the additional of a potential procedural team.

Based on the literature and experience, it was estimated that a Tier 1 provider onsite or as a tele-ICU provider could provide oversight care for 7–12 acutely/critically ill patients alone or possibly with the additional of a dedicated procedure team. Once this initial threshold is reached, Tier 2 providers will need to be added (each Tier 2 provider manages eight patients). With the addition of two Tier 2 providers, a Tier 1

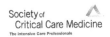

Tiered Staffing Strategy for Pandemic

Requiring Significant Mechanical Ventilation

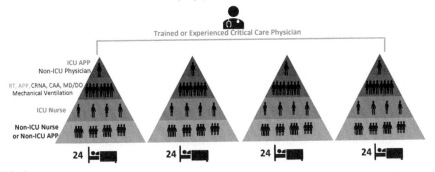

FIG. 2

A tired staffing model demonstrating how a small group of critical care experts working in concert with non-critical care providers can provide critical care to an expanded number of patients during a crisis. APP = advanced practice provider, CAA = certified anesthesiology assistant, CRNA = certified registered nurse anesthetist, DO = doctor of osteopathic medicine, MD = medical doctor, RT = respiratory therapist.

Reproduced with permission. Copyright © 2020 the Society of Critical Care Medicine.
https://www.ncbi.nlm.nih.gov/pmc/articles/PMC7314315/

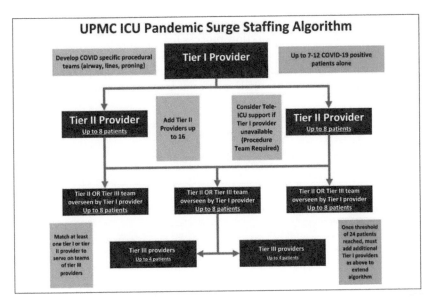

FIG. 3

A more detailed example of a tiered model for the expansion of critical care. Utilization of dedicated procedural teams for airway, central access, and proning is shown, allowing Tier 1 providers to be telemedicine and not on site. Tier 1 provider = critical care experts including telemedicine critical care; Tier 2 provider = providers with prior critical care training, experience, and skills (i.e., APP); Tier 3 = providers without previous critical care experience or skills. A separate classification as a "flex" tier would be those who might comprise a procedure team: providers with skill sets in intubation, bronchoscopy, central line insertion, arterial line insertion, prone positioning, but without bedside critical care expertise.

Reproduced with permission. Copyright © 2020 the Society of Critical Care Medicine.
https://www.ncbi.nlm.nih.gov/pmc/articles/PMC7314315/

provider could manage up to 16 patients. Once a threshold of 16 patients has been reached, an additional eight-patient team may need to be added to reach the highest threshold to manage 24 patients by a Tier 1 provider. Once the care of 16 patients is reached by the Tier 1 and 2 providers, it is recommended, if available, to add tele-ICU capabilities in addition to Tier 3 providers, who have no ICU experience, but can manage four patients each under the direction of the Tier 1 provider. This algorithm does not include resident or fellow trainees since there are many hospitals that do not have residents as part of their workforce. However, if trainees are available, they can be used as potential Tier 2 and 3 providers. Although this framework was originally developed by UPMC in response to the COVID-19 pandemic, this ICU provider staffing model can be applied for any response to increased ICU staffing demands for any disaster or mass critical care scenario.

At Geisinger, the critical care department and the biocontainment unit (BU) provided system expertise in the form of "site managers." The site managers taught just in time hands-on personal protective equipment (PPE) simulation for COVID-19 and educated redeployed employees to act as donning and doffing buddies in emergency departments and COVID units. As members of the BU, the site managers were also well trained in infection control and were deployed to hospitals, clinics, and nursing homes to help with infection control education. They also established and managed the workflow process for dedicated COVID units. Anesthesia, hospitalists, and surgeons were updated on the management of non-COVID critically ill patients in compacted classes based on commercially available professional societies courses. The eICU platform assists our hardest-hit hospitals (Fig. 4).

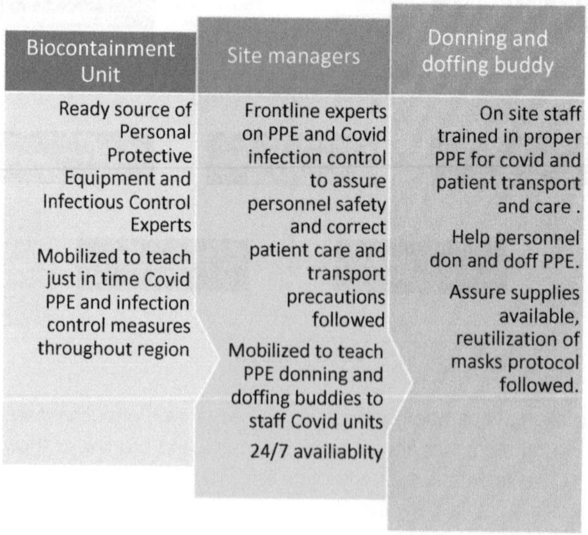

Biocontainment Unit	Site managers	Donning and doffing buddy
Ready source of Personal Protective Equipment and Infectious Control Experts	Frontline experts on PPE and Covid infection control to assure personnel safety and correct patient care and transport precautions followed	On site staff trained in proper PPE for covid and patient transport and care .
Mobilized to teach just in time Covid PPE and infection control measures throughout region	Mobilized to teach PPE donning and doffing buddies to staff Covid units	Help personnel don and doff PPE. Assure supplies available, reutilization of masks protocol followed.
	24/7 availiablity	

FIG. 4

Use of source experts to scale-up capability.

Space

At the system level, action plans should address the increased need for surge patient care area. Preparation and procedures should outline plans to increase capacity in current and surge states. The variability and dynamic nature of a disaster highlight the need for flexibility and fluidity in the organization. In real-time, patients must be managed and directed to the appropriate level of care. This coordinated effort must be collaborative and actively monitored.

In the pandemic's initial stages, COVID patients went to separate ICU and medical/surgical units. The conversion of existing ICU and med/surgical units into negative pressure rooms. The hospital's preparation supports the required capacity. As the rate of infections and hospital admission decreased, our leaders made conscious decisions to maintain all COVID patients in one unit. Our current structure cohorts all COVID patients (ICU vs non-ICU) for the hospital. That existing space is evaluated by leadership daily. Employees receive daily emails that graph current trends and patient volume. This indicator may be an early warning system for climbing infections and the potential need for increased capacity.

Once patients are out of the acute phase of illness, they transition to post-acute care. The patient's level of recovery determines appropriate placement. It can include skilled nursing facilities or home health. An adjunctive and flexible program at our institution is Geisinger at home. This program monitors patients at home with nursing visits and close follow-up during the post-acute care period. In the future, strengthening this outpatient network and mode of health-care delivery may reduce the need for hospital admission. The ability to offload intensive and resource-demanding care to the outpatient arena provides flexibility. In another way, innovation may transform future delivery of care.

How

a. Established "quality care" and evidence-based protocols are necessary to ensure basic practice standards. Multidisciplinary workgroups were assigned to tackle specific health-care areas and follow up-to-date evidence and emerging literature. Revisiting and revising past policies is essential to remain current and prepared for disaster. For instance, systemwide COVID-19 patient care guidelines were created by a multidisciplinary committee and updated weekly.

b. Innovation improves health-care delivery and resource utilization. During the pandemic, telehealth has received a significant boost in support. Our existing eICU platform provided support to our critical care colleagues at the most impacted locations. Additional telemedicine support in the outpatient setting allowed primary care providers to deliver preventative care. The innovation continues throughout the pandemic with alternative solutions to common problems.

Provider and family

The total impact of the virus is unknown, and health-care workers are not immune. Internal resilience often balances everyday stressors. However, the accumulation of additional burdens can disrupt the internal demand/resource paradigm. Without self-awareness, the transition from one level of functioning to another may progress to the point of dysfunction. Stress responses, such as increased irritability (flight), anxiety (flight), and stuck (freeze), should be recognized as warning signs. Often mental health is overlooked in times of disaster.

At Geisinger, we have a dedicated ICU psychologist who works as part of the care team, conducting evaluations, brief intervention, and assistance with managing psychological distress in patients and families. During the COVID pandemic, this psychologist continues to provide care, addressing delirium, acute anxiety, distress, and traumatic stress symptoms in hospitalized COVID-positive patients. She also provides an emotional support to patients' families via telephone, when distressed family members are identified by ICU staff.

It has been observed that COVID patients with higher severity of illness, often requiring higher levels of sedation, tend to experience increased delirium, agitation, delusional memories, and hallucinations during ICU stay. Furthermore, calls to distressed family members have been disproportionately made to families of younger, more severely ill patients, and those with more prolonged ICU stay.

In addition to patients and families, the ICU psychologist also regularly offers support to staff and frontline members of the care team. During the pandemic, this support has occurred both informally and formally. Informally, her presence in the COVID unit working among staff and inquiring about the well-being of care providers generally helps to increase the morale of unit staff. Formally, at the beginning of the pandemic, the psychologist assisted in facilitating the inception of a program designed to "care for the caregiver" or provide peer-to-peer support to hospital workers and staff, the Resilience in Stressful Events (RISE) program.[8] This program, designed at Johns Hopkins, is a confidential peer support initiative intended to provide in person brief psychological first aid and support to health-care personnel who have experienced stressful or distressing clinical events. RISE aims to decrease rates of burnout and second victim syndrome in health-care providers. This program is now used in more than 30 hospitals nationwide. At Geisinger, RISE, though initially planned to be implemented at the end of 2020 or early 2021, was expedited at the request of the critical care department to meet the rising stress of the COVID pandemic.

The continuum of COVID patient and family care does not end with hospital discharge. At Geisinger, many of these patients, based on the severity of illness, are offered participation in the post-ICU survivor clinic. Patients seen in the post-ICU clinic are regularly among the sickest patients treated in the ICU. During the initial clinic visit, patients, typically accompanied by a caregiver, are evaluated by the ICU psychologist, a critical care physician, and, for those with a history of documented delirium in the ICU, a neuropsychologist as well. At present, we have begun to see discharged COVID-positive patients and family members in the clinic. These patients appear to have some increase in post-ICU syndrome (PICS)—new or worsening impairment in physical, psychological, or cognitive health and functioning that occurs following critical illness and persists beyond discharge from the hospital.[9] We have observed our patients experiencing challenges with adjustment to ongoing respiratory and physical limitations (e.g., decreased lung capacity, shortness of breath, limited mobility, generalized weakness), anxiety and concern for future deterioration in health or reinfection with COVID, symptoms of posttraumatic stress disorder related to delusional memories associated with heavy sedation use (e.g., reexperiencing delusional memories in the form of flashbacks and nightmares), symptoms of depression, survivor guilt, anger, and, in one patient, ongoing inattention and visual hallucinations despite otherwise normal recovery. We have referred some of these patients for ongoing treatment with psychologists or further evaluation with neuropsychology, along with follow-up care for physical concerns. Caregivers of COVID-19 patients have also reported psychological distress associated with isolation during the hospital stay, perception of the slow recovery of loved ones, and anxiety associated with the health concerns.

Patients with COVID-19 are at increased risk of delirium due to multiple proposed mechanisms and pathways associated with this virus.[10] Higher rates of delirium during ICU admission increases the likelihood that COVID patients will have ongoing needs, including PICS following hospital discharge. Also, isolation associated with restrictions in visitation policies and hospitals and post-acute care settings, and higher rates of illness severity and complication, increase the risk that family members and caregivers of COVID patients will experience long-standing psychological distress (i.e., PICS-families [PICS-F]). Thus a post-ICU clinic, like ours at Geisinger, is a vital part of assessing and addressing the ongoing needs of COVID-positive patients and families following hospital discharge.

Other disaster care during COVID-19—Experiences from the front line

Other disasters, both natural and human made, will occur during a global pandemic—additional states of disaster stress a tenuous health-care delivery system. Disasters, in conjunction with COVID, will present unique and unprecedented challenges. Health-care institutions should review their emergency operations plan to incorporate COVID mitigation strategies that apply during events that cause an influx of patients. Recent examples include Hurricane Laura and the West Coast wildfires. A state of emergency and disaster, if appropriately prepared, can be managed successfully.

1. Natural disasters

    Natural disasters such as hurricanes, floods, earthquakes, wildfires, tornadoes, tsunamis, volcanic eruptions, etc. continue to occur globally. Given modern advances, some of these events now have an advanced warning from minutes to days in advance. The large-scale geographical impact of events can displace a large number of people. Displaced people will need shelter; some people will have complex medical needs or comorbidities. Shelter layout requires planning and needs evaluation in the era of COVID.

Forcing social distancing can be accomplished by limiting and distancing the number of cots placed in a shelter. Utilizing additional areas for the housing of displaced persons, like hotels, would be preferred as it is more accessible to cohort those screening positive for COVID exposure and symptoms. Cohorts of families in shelters also assist in social distancing among other occupants. The health-care system may assist with daily patient screening in shelters (temperature screening and COVID symptom questions). Health-care staff may also be displaced and could require housing assistance. At our institution, call rooms and off-campus housing were open to any staff who required isolation or quarantine. If able, health-care facilities should ascertain where all patients are presenting from and where they are lodging.

Contact tracing and early mitigation are essential for COVID-positive patients. Natural disasters can cause an initial influx of patients from injuries due to the event. If the infrastructure is damaged, patients can overwhelm functioning hospitals or clinics by presenting with minor illnesses or injuries; in the recovery phase, patients may seek medication refills and treatment for cellulitis, insect bites, sprains/strains, laceration repairs, etc.

2. Human-made disasters

Human-made disasters such as active killer events, events involving chemicals, explosions, transportation accidents, acts of terrorism, etc. continue to present systemic challenges. These events are usually chaotic, unpredictable, and can result in many patients presenting to hospitals to seek treatment. A majority of patients may self-present to a hospital for treatment; emergency medical services agencies, especially in rural settings, may be overtaxed by the volume of patients at the scene.

Due to the acuity and volume of patients presenting to a hospital during the initial phase of the disaster, it may be impossible to screen all patients for COVID signs and symptoms. Emergent and aerosolizing procedures may be required for multiple patients. In most instances, patients with chemical exposure will need decontamination before entering the hospital. Attempts to distance and to apply universal masking to patients in decontamination lines may not be feasible. Wet decontamination is accomplished with copious amounts of water and soap. The goal is to decontaminate as many patients in a short period effectively and limits sanitizing in between patients.

3. Mitigation strategies

In the event of a disaster, these mitigation strategies may assist in curbing and containing the spread of COVID. Depending upon the situation, some of these strategies are relatively easier to implement and may already be in place before a disaster occurs. It is imperative that even in a disaster, we do not forget the basics—handwashing, cleaning equipment/surfaces, and proper donning/doffing of PPE; staff safety will always take precedence. Including COVID mitigation strategies in disaster planning and preparedness is essential. Testing these strategies before an actual disaster will assist in finding deficiencies that can be improved upon and will make staff more comfortable and familiar with the disaster plan.

- Universal source control should be implemented by masking all individuals presenting to a hospital or shelter. Hospitals would need to ensure that an adequate supply of masks are available for distribution as there will be an increase in demand.
- If possible, all individuals should undergo screening before entry into the hospital. Screening would consist of temperature checks, questions to identify COVID symptoms, and questions to identify potential exposure to COVID or those with COVID symptoms. Patients requiring lifesaving interventions, higher acuity patients, and those who are not capable of adequately answering questions may not be screened. If space allows, cohort patients with positive COVID signs/symptoms into a separate isolation area and positive COVID exposure into a separate quarantine area.
- Consider having all staff providing direct patient care wear an N95 mask with eye protection (or powered air-purifying respirators, if available, for those who failed fit testing) for all patient encounters.
- COVID testing is already challenging, and availability/laboratory capacity is stretched further during a disaster.
- Increasing the opportunity to perform hygiene is paramount. Adding or increasing the quantity of alcohol-based hand rub in patient care areas and areas where people may be gathering can increase compliance with sanitizing hands. If water supply has been compromised, the addition of portable handwashing stations would be highly beneficial.
- The frequency of sanitizing patient care areas, high-touch surfaces, communal bathroom/shower areas, and sleeping areas should be increased.
- Displaced hospital staff may need lodging in the event their homes were damaged or destroyed. Locating lodging space for displaced staff on the hospital campus is beneficial. Keeping the same staff from different shifts assigned to the same individual sleeping area would reduce the number of people exposed if a staff member becomes positive; having a sign-in log would help track staff in an exposure. Cleaning of the lodging area should be performed between shifts.

References

1. Hossain T, Ghazipura M, Dichter JR. Intensive care role in disaster management critical care clinics. *Crit Care Clin*. 2019;35(4):535–550.
2. National Health Security Preparedness Index. *Update National Health Security Index*. Robert Wood Johnson Foundation; 2019. Available at: https//nhspi.org/. Accessed 10 September 2020.

3. Hardy S, Fattah S, Wisborg T, Raatiniemi L, Staff T, Rehn M. Systematic reporting to improve the emergency medical response to major incidents: a pilot study. *BMC Emerg Med.* 2018;18(1):4. https://www.ncbi.nlm.nih.gov/pubmed/29368642. https://doi.org/10.1186/s12873-018-0153-x.
4. Toerper MF, Kelen GD, Sauer LM, Bayram JD, Catlett C, Levin S. Hospital surge capacity: a web-based simulation tool for emergency planners. *Disaster Med Public Health Prep.* 2018;12(4):513–522. https://www.ncbi.nlm.nih.gov/pubmed/29041994. https://doi.org/10.1017/dmp.2017.93.
5. Manley WG, Furbee PM, Coben JH, et al. Realities of disaster preparedness in rural hospitals. *Disaster Manag Response.* 2006;4(3):80–87. https://doi.org/10.1016/j.dmr.2006.05.001.
6. Society of Critical Care Medicine. *ICU Readiness Assessment: We Are Not Prepared for COVID-19*; 2020. Available at: https://www.sccm.org/getattachment/Blog/April-2020/ICU-Readiness-Assessment-We-AreNot-Prepared-for/COVID-19-Readiness-Assessment-Survey-SCCM.pdf?lang=en-US.
7. Harris GH, Baldisseri MR, Reynolds BR, Orsino AS, Sackrowitz R, Bishop JM. Design for Implementation of a system-level ICU pandemic surge staffing plan. *Crit Care Explor.* 2020;2(6):e0136. https://doi.org/10.1097/CCE.0000000000000136.
8. Edrees H, Connors C, Paine L, et al. Implementing the RISE second victim support programme at the Johns Hopkins Hospital: a case study. *BMJ Open.* 2016;6. https://doi.org/10.1136/bmjopen-2016-011708, e011708. 27694486.
9. Needham DM, Davidson J, Cohen H, et al. Improving long-term outcomes after discharge from intensive care unit: report from a stakeholders' conference. *Crit Care Med.* 2012;40:502–509.
10. Kotfis K, Williams Roberson S, Wilson JE, Dabrowski W, Pun BT, Ely EW. COVID-19: ICU delirium management during SARS-CoV-2 pandemic. *Crit Care.* 2020;24(1):1–176. https://doi.org/10.1186/s13054-020-02882-x.

My experience with the novel coronavirus: As doctor and patient

3

Deena Lynch

Brisbane, QLD, Australia

"She's young," I thought to myself one night as the intensive care physician on call in the hospital. I had been called to evaluate a patient in her thirties who had recently been confirmed as having contracted the (then) novel coronavirus. She possessed none of the attributes that medical school and residency teachings suggest are typical risk factors for the ravaging lung injury demonstrated on computed tomography and X-ray of her chest.

"Do you, or have you smoked cigarettes?" I asked.

"No."

"Any illicit drugs?"

"No," she answered, as if knowingly that I was searching for an etiologic explanation for her presentation.

She'd been placed on a form of supplemental oxygen that effectively delivers 100% oxygen through a mask. I took it off to see where her measured oxygen levels would taper off to. Almost immediately, the bedside monitor emitted its ominous alarm indicating plummeting oxygen levels. She remained calm; her husband stood by her with a persistent look of concern. I replaced the mask and waited for oxygen levels to normalize.

"You're pretty dependent on this oxygen. For the next step, we're going to need to take is to place you on a ventilator with a breathing tube to support you. It means you're going to need to come to the intensive care unit (ICU)," I said.

"Are you sure I need something that's aggressive, doctor?" she asked.

"No. I'm not sure. But I've never seen healthy lungs get this bad this quickly and I don't know the direction you're ultimately headed," is what went through my head.

"The rate of your lung injury progression and your need for 100% oxygen suggests that you're going to need significant ventilatory support in the pretty near future," is what came out of my mouth instead. She ultimately agreed to endotracheal intubation and mechanical ventilatory support while receiving what we thought were the right remedies for this new and novel coronavirus.

She was one of the first of hundreds that would present to our hospital and that I would treat and of thousands that would go on to confound medical expertise and plunge the world as we knew it into unprecedented social, economic, and political turmoil.

COVID-19 Pandemic. https://doi.org/10.1016/B978-0-323-82860-4.00014-8

Colleagues and I were preparing on the front lines of this pandemic as I watched the devastation wash over my old residency training stomping grounds in Elmhurst Hospital Center (a Level 1 trauma county hospital caring for the Queens, New York community of the same name) from my newest professional perch in a large hospital in Miami, Florida. We devised plans here at Baptist Hospital of Miami's Critical Care Department for provision of personal protective equipment, enlisted the help of other physician specialties in the event that virus caseloads overwhelmed our already stretched Critical Care team and outlined schema to safely place breathing tubes into trachea expelling potentially deadly virus while ensuring our own safety.

And then we braced for impact. We would receive daily updates of case numbers and clinical tidbits outlining state-of-the-art diagnostic and therapeutic strategies. We would don and doff cumbersome protective suits to exact specifications of sealing at the neck and wrists. Physicians and nurses all emerged drenched in sweat after rendering care beneath layers of protective equipment necessitating several changes of scrubs each shift. We would read of others' experiences and the crushing psychological and emotional toll to care for someone that you could not touch and had to veritably scream at to communicate through such enclosed protection. I had not consumed much of this content through the general news media, whom I would long ago decided was too sensationalistic to view. This was all delivered from the world's newest medium, social media. Colleagues and friends would proclaim their own experiences and challenges and many of them rivaled my own in concern, sadness, and overwhelm.

In an effort to bolster our capacity, we enlisted more nursing staff sourced from other clinical departments (medical wards, emergency department, even pediatrics) as well as from temporary travel nursing agencies. Clinical care was rendered not only from the bedside but also from the glass-enclosed doorways of each ICU room; intravenous pumps generally placed at the immediate bedside of the patient were relegated to outside their rooms with eight-to-ten feet of extension tubing running to the patient. To the lay person observer, walking into our ICU caring for patients debilitated with COVID-19, it would appear as though our patients were ostensibly encapsulated in glass pods similar to movie scenes depicting alien life-forms being kept in secret government compounds. They were being cared for by staff in eye protection, masks and non permeable suits, dialing pump settings at each room's doorway. Compounding this surreal scene was our need for placing patients on their stomachs (known as "prone position") to help optimize their lungs for oxygenation and ventilation and obscuring their faces.

All of these measures were taken to care for some of the sickest patients I have ever seen, while protecting the caregivers. As a specialist in Emergency Medicine and Critical Care Medicine, one of the most frightening scenarios encountered is the lungs of a patient that cannot be oxygenated or ventilated, despite the most aggressive measures. It is a case that practitioners and educators of critical illness prepare for and are in constant fear of.

Circumstances like these have not been recounted in recent memory and for those of us subject to them, especially those accustomed to acuity of less severity, we were tested to our physical, psychological, and emotional limits. Skin breakdown was evident over areas under consecutive hours of pressure on caregivers' faces, only to be framed with the solemn eyes of someone who has fought to maintain a person's basic vital functions like adequate blood pressure to live or oxygen levels to survive. Some left, unable to reconcile the extent of disease, and the injury that our medical interventions caused with the seemingly unstoppable progression of multi-organ failure and eventual death.

For those of us that remained, we were lauded as heroic and brave. It did not feel that way. Despite the multitude of accolades doled out for those in medical scrubs, from evening noise by pot and pan banging in salutation, to murals on buildings, what went unnoticed was the overwhelming sense of futility and frustration at trying to understand a yet unknown disease process while watching its progression ravage human beings regardless of what we did.

Yet, in this haze, there was good. In spite of national division and derision about this viral pandemic, in our microsphere of Critical Care at Baptist Hospital of Miami, the exhausted, determined, facially scarred care providers became galvanized. Spirits came together in unity over what seemed to be an abundance of donated food (lots of pizza). With increasing familiarity of the natural history of critically afflicted patients by the novel coronavirus, we began to see outcomes in patients that we were proud of.

An initial significant test of our mettle came when several cruise ships that had been denied port at other countries were accepted to the Port of Miami. Several large hospitals in the area (including the Baptist Hospital) had agreed to take patients off of these cruise ships, some of which had been at sea for weeks. We received notice and again, braced for impact. Estimates of patient caseloads varied wildly. Patients included travelers as well as staff from these cruise ships. Their ages ranged from staff in their 1930s to travelers older than 75 years old. There was no compass with which to effectively prognosticate; we would support their cardiopulmonary systems day by day and could only see how things would go. But, day by day, those who appeared destined to not survive began to improve. Ventilatory support requirements would decrease. Blood pressure support would decrease. Their vital functions began to return. Ultimately, we repatriated many of these patients to their origin nations, including a young 40-year-old male to his family in the Philippines, a gentleman in his 1970s back to his wife in New Zealand and another to his home country of the United Kingdom. A most gratifying case was one of a 40-year-old gentleman that had recently been seen by an infectious disease colleague of mine in her outpatient clinic after getting home from hospitalization in the ICU because he had burning pain on urination; a benign complaint that I was happy to hear he had lived to complain about at all.

It was during this relatively elated time that I began to feel increasing fatigue and generalized weakness overall. I had suspected it was simply working exhausting hours with weeks that regularly exceeded 80 h. I checked my temperature at home. 103.5 F. No, it could not be. I checked again; it was real. I went to the emergency room where a rapid nasopharyngeal swab confirmed my worst fear. I had contracted the novel coronavirus. And worse, with symptoms, I was developing the COVID-19 syndrome. I knew what was coming. Visions of those I had cared for; those in medical comas on mechanical ventilators, paralyzed, sedated, and placed in prone positions to optimize their ever so frail lungs. And the resultant death. I had never had to truly face my own mortality with the fund of knowledge and understanding that I had with this disease.

The typical disease trajectory for those with competent immune systems goes like this: first, general malaise with fever, Maybe a cough, body aches, decreased appetite and loss of sense of taste and smell. Those less fortunate may develop serious conditions like stroke or heart attack from occlusion of their respective arteries, cerebral, or coronary. These are the usual signs and symptoms for the first 3–6 days.

Then, things get scary. If the lungs are going to feature prominently, they will declare at around 3–5 days in. Breathing will become more difficult. Oxygen levels will plummet. I was unable to get to the bathroom or kitchen in my condominium unit without becoming winded. Measured oxygen levels read as low as 88% (normal is around 100%). I should have presented to hospital, but like every doctor that makes for a terrible patient, I waited. Luckily for me, things began to improve beginning on the fifth day, and I was without fever or symptoms by 10 days after diagnosis.

I now live my life with a renewed sense of vulnerability and realization of my own mortality. And having cared for patients clinging to life, some who lost that battle and some who won, I also live my life with new humility. We train as medical doctors to heal and comfort. We have been hurtled into a chapter in history that tests that very resilience. To pronounce previously, vivacious people dead after attempting extreme lifesaving measures is difficult enough. To do it within the context of an unknown pathophysiologic adversary in repeated fashion will take some of us to dark places in our own psychological recesses. It was not long after I resumed caring for COVID-19 patients that I heard the name Dr. Lorna Breen. She was a fellow emergency physician who claimed her own life after describing scenes, she observed of the toll this novel coronavirus took on her patients.

This story lifted the lid on another morbidity and mortality toll in addition to the many ill patients stricken with the disease; the mental health and wellness of the people caring for them. We operate in a domain of great stress, high stakes, and easy criticism from any not immediately beside us. The intention is pure; we want to save lives and cure disease. But when that intention is tested and we are unable to carry this purpose to bear, the helplessness experienced by such empowered professional individuals can be crippling. I say this not to incite sympathy but to realize that, while some of us will deny it, we all need the unity and support of society for all of us to endure this. To divide this pandemic on the basis of misinformation, lack of government leadership or guidance will only serve to fracture the institution of the sick from the nonbelievers further. Please believe me, I have seen it. We just want the critically ill to get better and to return them to the loved ones that weren't allowed to visit them and, failing that, we need to be able to cope with our own perceived failures when we cannot do so. And we cannot do that without your support and understanding.

This novel coronavirus has killed individuals of all ages, socioeconomic status, gender, and has similarly brought the world's civilizations to our collective knees. We no longer travel by plane in the same fashion that we did, we are wary of anyone with a slight cough, innumerable households worry where they will find money to eat. But in this time that will be marked as one of the darkest in modern history, we have a chance now to reunite and join as global citizens to protect each other, and most importantly, respect each other. If it's possible for the provider teams of nurse, physicians, and all other staff to galvanize in a surreal war zone of human suffering and death while still saving lives in the face of a ghost adversary at Baptist Hospital Critical Care, then surely it can be extrapolated to unity of citizens of a society facing one of the largest pandemics in recent history.

COVID-19: A family's perspective

4

María Cruz Martín Delgado

Intensive Care Unit, Hospital Universitario de Torrejón, Madrid, Spain Universidad Francisco de Vitoria, Madrid, Spain

The emergence of a new virus of the Coronaviridae family, called severe acute respiratory syndrome coronavirus 2 (SARS-CoV-2) which was detected for the first time in December 2019 in Wuhan (China), has led to the definition of a new disease known as coronavirus disease 2019 (COVID-19).[1]

Up to date, this condition has affected over 90 million patients in 188 countries around the world, with almost 2 million deaths.[2] In its more severe presentation, the SARS-CoV-2 infection causes acute respiratory failure that requires mechanical ventilation in a high proportion of cases.[3–6] In Spain, more than 11,500 persons have been admitted to intensive care units (ICU) due to COVID-19, typically with prolonged stays and a high percentage of mortality.[6]

The characteristics of this highly contagious and lethal disease have compelled governments to adopt extraordinary measures in most countries, including a declaration of a state of emergency, the general confinement of the population, the encouragement of social distancing, the isolation of patients and their close contacts, and the implementation of restrictive visiting policies both in social and health-care facilities.[7–9]

Although these measures have demonstrated to be effective to flatten the epidemic curve, they have resulted in radical changes in social and health-care practices.[10] These new policies have caused patients and their relatives to suffer through the disease in isolation and family separation, even in challenging and unique moments such as end-of-life events. These and other factors have altered the family unit and its dynamics during the pandemic.

Post-intensive care syndrome (PICS-P) affects many critically ill patients (30%–50%). It encompasses physical (mainly respiratory and neuromuscular systems), cognitive (memory and attention deficits), and psychological [depression, anxiety, stress, and post-traumatic stress disorder (PTSD)] sequelae that appear after discharge from the ICU and impact negatively their quality of life.[11]

This syndrome also affects family members (PICS-F), a vulnerable population that suffers negative physical, psychological, and social effects which also lead to a deterioration in their quality of life.[12]

41

COVID-19 Pandemic. https://doi.org/10.1016/B978-0-323-82860-4.00017-3

Data from several studies show a high prevalence of anxiety (73%),[13] depression (35%),[14] PTSD (56%),[15] and complicated grief (52%)[16] in relatives of ICU patients.[17] These sequelae can be long lasting. The Randomized Evaluation of COVID-19 Therapy (RECOVER) study revealed that 16% of relatives had not reduced their level of depression 1 year after the discharge of their patients.[17]

They also exhibit physical symptoms such as fatigue and health risk behaviors such as sleep disturbances, insufficient rest, sedentarism, unbalanced diets, and non-compliance with medical treatment. The burden of caring for a patient who has been severely ill can affect personal aspects of the family's life plans and their social and professional relationships; it also tends to foster family conflicts.[18]

A study assessing the components of PICS-P's impact on the family members who care for the patient found a low burden level in 34.5% of caregivers and a moderate–high level in 15.5% of caregivers. The presence of psychological components of the PICS-P (anxiety and depression) 3 months after discharge from the ICU affected negatively the burden of the caregiver. Neither physical sequelae nor other measured variables had any significant impact of the caregiver burden.[19]

The Society of Critical Care Medicine assumes the concept of family as defined by the patient, or in the case of minors (who have no legal decision-making capacity) by their surrogates.[20] In this context, "family" may or may not be actually related to the patient. Rather, they are supportive individuals with whom the patient has a meaningful relationship.

A person's admission to the ICU causes an alteration of the family structure and function, creating a series of disorders and feelings and an overall experience that is almost always described as traumatic. When this occurs, family members must deal with emotional, cognitive, and social stressors that generate feelings of shock, uncertainty, denial, anger, despair, hope, guilt, anxiety, and fear of the patient's death. If the stressors exceed the family's coping ability to handle the situation (and in many cases the family has limited adaptation resources or a lack of habit to use them), they become subjects in need of care.[21]

The primary needs of families who have a patient in the ICU include (1) receiving truthful and understandable information about the patient's status; (2) assurance that their loved one is not alone and that as family members they can reassure, protect, and support their patient; (3) receiving some hope about the possibility of recovery or at least, in the event of a hopeless situation, the assurance of a painless and dignified death; (4) the perception that their patient is well cared for; and (5) the perception that the professionals caring for their relative have the necessary skills to perform an effective job.

If those needs are met, it will bring the family relief from anxiety and some degree of comfort.[22]

The concept of person-centered medicine recognizes not only the needs of the patient but also the needs of the family members. This leads to the consideration that families cannot be viewed as mere "visitors"; indeed, they constitute an indissoluble bond that makes them relevant actors in the face of critical illness. Family-centered care recognizes the paramount role of the family in the patient's recovery. It describes the health-care team's responsibility to provide support to critically ill patient's families, to be respectful, and respond adequately to each family's individual needs and values.

The "Guidelines for Family-Centered Care in the Neonatal, Pediatric, and Adult ICU"[23] published in 2016 established a series of recommendations based on the scientific evidence to optimize the support of ICU patients' families. These recommendations include the family's presence in the ICU, family support, open communication with the family, inclusion of specific consultants in the team such as specialists in ethics, psychological support or aspects related to the organization, and structure of these units.

The strategies to detect and prevent PICS require a structured and early multidisciplinary approach to the critical patient's admission. The measures should allow for the detection of risk factors not only for the development of sequelae both in the patient and in the family members. There are many initiatives and recommendations established to reduce PICS-P's appearance which are gradually being implemented in ICUs as standard policies.

The "ICU liberation"[24] concept is a quality improvement initiative based on the implementation of the ABCDEF set of evidence-based measures, which has shown that, when applied comprehensively, it improves outcomes and reduces the incidence of PICS. Pain control, adequate sedation, delirium management, keeping patients awake and breathing spontaneously, early mobilization, and family's early involvement and participation all have shown to increase patient's survival and to reduce sequelae in patients and their families after discharge from the ICU.[25]

There is not much scientific evidence available on interventions to reduce PICS-F. A systematic review shows that proactive communication and adequate information are essential elements to ameliorate the sequelae of critically ill patient families.[26] Certain interventions can actually worsen the situation, for example, meetings held by external palliative teams without ICU professionals' participation. On the other hand, actions such as sending a condolence letter after a patient's death could decrease the incidence of PTSD.[27,28]

In recent years, humanization of intensive care units has advanced significantly through different initiatives, such as the HU-CI project.[29] This international and multidisciplinary project spearheads a change in the paradigm of critical patient care (following eight different guidelines), offering a frame of reference for humanized intensive care.[30] The implementation of these initiatives has led to opening the doors of ICUs for extended hours to family members, to allow the presence and active participation of the families in the care and even specific procedures of their patient, to form "families," to communicate openly and more freely with the patient and the professionals in the attending team, and for the families to be present at the end-of-life events.[31]

The recent pandemic has put the health system in check and has shaken many of these policies that were being gradually implemented in many units. On the other hand, it has highlighted the importance of preserving these directive strategies. The pandemic has also unveiled the emotional effect that this disease has brought to patients, families, and health-care professionals. The separation of the most severely ill patients from their families shows the cruelest side of the pandemic.[32]

During this time, we have seen how patients remain isolated from their families, increasing their fears and anxiety in the face of a severe illness that could potentially lead to death and of the loneliness and isolation during their extended admission to the ICU. Families have had to live with the uncertainty of what was happening in these units, while the media showed saturated units and insufficient resources to care for all seriously ill patients.

The communication and decision-making process have been hampered by the reduction of direct contact with professionals, regarding essential aspects such as the decision to admit somebody to the ICU or the limitation of life-support treatment. Therapeutic decisions have been made regarding specific treatments, many of them as "off-label", compassionate (if unproven) use, or the inclusion of clinical trials with great uncertainty not only from the clinical point of view but also from the decision-making process as well.[33]

Finally, many families have not been able to accompany their loved ones at the end-of-life[34] events and have even had difficulties to say goodbye, to perform the usual rituals, or to dispose of the body after the demise of the patient. All of this suggests a significant impact on the incidence of PICS-P on those who have over-come the disease, but also of PICS-F, particularly in families of deceased patients.[35]

Health professionals have experienced extraordinary situations in which the high demand for care, often accompanied by a shortage or scarcity of resources, has led to the health system's saturation. In response, intensive care teams have expanded their units structurally, occupying new spaces and taking in other professionals who normally do not attend critically ill patients, and even using equipment that is not always adequate.[36] Meanwhile, the lack or shortage of proper personal protective equipment (PPE) has exposed health professionals to the risk of infecting themselves and their families. The problem intensifies due to the strenuous, prolonged, and exhausting shifts, the reduction of the workforce, the unavailability of diagnostic tests, and the realization that the quality of care being provided is not always adequate.[37]

The emotional suffering that the restricted visitation policy has infringed on health professionals is known to be high. Generally, the population has always recognized the timely and effective response of health-care teams, and now, those teams are seeking and finding new ways to overcome the limitations set by the pandemic itself. Health-care professionals have become innovative and are offering tools such as telecommunications and videoconferencing, in an attempt to shorten the distance between patients and their families. This situation is and will continue to impact health professionals who are at high risk of suffering burnout, moral distress, compassion fatigue, and PTSD.[38]

Restricted visitation policies

The COVID-19 pandemic response has included drastic restrictions on hospital visits with the well-intentioned goal of social distancing to reduce the risk of infection.[39] These decisions, adopted in a generalized way and sometimes with absolute prohibitions, could be considered ethical, based on prioritizing public health[40] protection. Unfortunately, by their very nature, they undoubtedly prevent the delivery of humanized care focused on the family, especially in the most challenging situations and at the end-of-life events. These restrictive policies have been implemented abruptly, and in many cases, without the input of key stakeholders including the patients themselves, their families, and the health-care professionals. A critical reflection has led to alternative options in which greater importance is given to the accepted normative rights of patients (such as the right to be accompanied, the right to have spiritual or religious support) and questions if the limitations imposed can be of such intensity that become a de facto deprivation of these rights.[41]

Restrictions on family presence should not undermine the principles of family-centered care, and for this, it is necessary to adapt tools and procedures to the new context. The goals of this type of care during the COVID-19 pandemic should be geared towards[1] respecting the family's role as team members,[2] collaboration between family members and health-care professionals, and[3] maintaining family integrity.[42]

As an alternative to the visit limitations, many units have developed support systems and initiatives using technology to minimize isolation and to bring families closer to their hospitalized patient. The use of these devices has led to ethical and legal debates over the availability and inequity of these resources and data privacy protection. Regulations should be established to protect patients and their families' rights and to reduce the risk of legal suits to health-care professionals.

The positive experience of some ICUs with more flexible visitation policies should be considered in the future to avoid, as far as possible, the effects derived from strict isolation. As Andrist et al.[8] established, we should not allow severe restrictions to become routine in the ICU as it weakens the current trend of humanization. His pediatric ICU experience shows how it is possible to adapt the rules to facilitate more open and flexible visits in a safe way. These authors remind us that all administrative measures have exceptions for certain essential activities. Accompanying patients, especially as an end-of-life event, is an important activity supported by ethical and legal international frameworks. There can be no reason for a patient to die alone. For this, adequate communication plan is necessary to transparently inform the family how these visits will be carried out and to avoid conflicts, allowing the family to understand the reason for the restrictions imposed. Having specific written protocols in which these policies are clearly explained can facilitate the implementations of the visits. The protocols must be dynamically adapted as the pandemics evolve.

Certain measures can help to adopt less restrictive policies while minimizing the infection risk for everybody. It is essential to have suitable PPEs for families, to ensure adequate training in the use of the equipment, and to adapt procedures to the structural characteristics of each unit and its resources. Specific policies should also be considered for critical patients admitted to non-COVID-19 units, where the restrictions are limited to monitoring for the disease. In cases where visits are considered a limited resource, it may be necessary for independent multidisciplinary bodies to allocate those resources. Recommendations have been proposed to maintain the connection of COVID-19 patients with their families, which help to reduce the negative impact of restricting visits.[43]

The family's presence and company can go hand in hand with the family's participation and involvement in the care of their patient. Even though this participation is considered a voluntary individualized process that develops progressively, it should be guided by the health-care professionals. Due to the pandemic, this participation in caregiving has no longer been possible due to visit limitation and saturation of health-care facilities; many health-care teams are overwhelmed and have no time to do necessary preparations.

Recently, the family's presence during specific procedures[44,45] such as cardiopulmonary resuscitation has shown beneficial effects, as long as it is performed in appropriate settings. Interventions like these, still limited in many units, have been questioned during the pandemic, especially in procedures with a high risk of infection or in which resources and equipment are scarce. Alternative measures such as tele-accompaniment, quarantine imposition, and even pet's[46] company have been proposed.

Other aspects related to family care has been the need to transfer patients to other hospitals (which may be located in a different geographic area) to optimize the use of resources.[47] Factors like distance, limitation of traveling and even communicating with the family, and the epidemic controls imposed on traveling all contribute to increase the family's suffering and emotional trauma. In this context, prior and open communication with the family is recommended to explain clearly the reasons for the transfer, the patient's final destination, and the ways to keep in contact with the new facility (including a phone contact number).

Communicating with the family

The appearance of PICS-F has been related to ineffective communication between the health-care teams and the family, which naturally influences the family's perception and the experience during and after their relative has been in the ICU.[48] Lack of or inadequate information is related to the development of PTSD.[49] Adequate timely information and open communication with family members are essential aspects of the care in critically ill patients, especially on the occasions when the family takes the decision-making role on behalf of a patient who may not be able to do so on its own. In those instances, it is vital to provide information from the beginning and update the family regularly, especially when changes in the treatment are expected.

In the context of the pandemic, there are diverse activities that can be implemented to improve communication with the family: question and answer meetings, general information about the health-care process, a visit to the ICU to show the family what is actually done there (including interventions such as mechanical ventilation or tracheostomy),[50] information about PICS and its components such as delirium or the emotional response to being discharged from the ICU),[51] and the setting of a system to send and receive texts, messages, and videos all with the goal to bring closer the family to their patient.

Synchronous communication refers to communication between the patient and his/her family or the family and the health-care team. Structured communication must be carried out proactively, daily and, in situations that demand it due to their severity. Families must know the established communication plan either in person or online to reduce the uncertainty and stress generated by waiting for a call. Communicating with the patient and the family includes not just getting clinical information about the patient but also serving as a form of therapy by providing assurance, comfort, and a measure of dignity. Moreover, it can help to get to know the patient better as an individual and to know his preferences to help the family to take the best decisions possible regarding the patient's therapy, particularly in complex situations. Also, it can help to set therapeutic goals based not only on the clinical progress of the patient but also on his preferences too.[52]

During the pandemic, many initiatives have been promoted by different associations and by the health-care teams to bring families and patients closer using calls and videoconferencing.[53] The latter facilitates emotional ties through facial expressions and nonverbal communication. To achieve effective communication, the technology itself is not enough; specific training for health-care professionals to appropriately use the gadgets and guidelines to ensure their effectiveness are necessary.

End-of-life event

The end of life constitutes a traumatic event for families of patients who die during their stay in the ICU, particularly in those surrogates of patients who are incapable of taking their own decisions. The presence of the family and an adequate communication with the health-care team are essential, the more so in end-of-life care situations.[16] There is evidence that families who cannot say farewell to a relative present a higher risk of complicated grief. At the end of life of a patient, the physical, psychological, emotional, and spiritual needs of the family must be addressed, informing them of the changes in care as the disease evolves and tailoring the treatment of the patient to his preferences and those of the family.

Family's accompaniment in moments like this constitute a right in which no person shall be deprived of his life. Consequently, restrictive policies must be flexible as much as possible, allowing the family to say their farewell. Of course, to facilitate these visits require appropriate PPE as well as to train and prepare the family and to provide them with an adequate space that allows for intimacy and privacy. Whenever that is not possible, distance accompaniment by means of teleconferencing must be encouraged, always following the family's preferences. Honestly, open communication can help families[54] to understand better the death process and to deal and prevent pathological states of grief. Facilitating emotional support to the family by the mental health specialists can prevent psychological sequelae and ensure mental well-being. There are established recommendations and tools that help families and health-care professionals to deal with grief, including quality communication, advance planning and writing of a will, and self-care.[55]

Conclusion

The restrictions imposed by the COVID-19 pandemic should not decrease the family-centered care. In fact, in these circumstances, care for the family has become even more relevant. The health-care system and its professionals must adapt the established strategies to the new circumstances to become innovative through the use of technology keeping humanization of care as a key element to offer the best possible care to patients and their families. All of this will yield better results in health care and will help to reduce the prevalence of PICS both in patients and their families.

Finally, these initiatives can also have a positive impact on the health-care professionals, decreasing emotional suffering, compassion fatigue, and burnout.

References

1. Munster VJ, Koopmans M, van Doremalen N, van Riel D, de Wit E. A novel coronavirus emerging in China - key questions for impact assessment. *N Engl J Med.* 2020;382 (8):692–694.
2. https://coronavirus.jhu.edu/map.html Accessed 6 July 2020.
3. Wu Z, Mc Googan JM. Characteristics of and important lessons from the coronavirus disease 2019 (COVID-19) outbreak in China: summary of a report of 72 314 cases from the Chinese Center for Disease Control and Prevention [published online February 24, 2020]. JAMA doi:https://doi.org/10.1001/jama.2020.2648.
4. Huang C, Wang Y, Li X, et al. Clinical features of patients infected with 2019 novel coronavirus in Wuhan, China. *Lancet.* 2020;395(10223):497–506. https://doi.org/10.1016/S0140-6736(20)30183-5.
5. Wang D, Hu B, Hu C, et al. Clinical characteristics of 138 hospitalized patients with 2019 novel coronavirus–infected pneumonia in Wuhan. *JAMA.* 2020;323(11):1061–1069. https://doi.org/10.1001/jama.2020.1585.
6. https://www.mscbs.gob.es/profesionales/saludPublica/ccayes/alertasActual/nCov-China/documentos/Actualizacion_154_COVID-19.pdf Accessed 6 July 2020.

7. Nussbaumer-Streit B, Mayr V, Dobrescu AI, et al. Quarantine alone or in combination with other public health measures to control COVID-19: a rapid review. *Cochrane Database Syst Rev.* 2020;4(4):CD013574. Published 2020 Apr 8 https://doi.org/10.1002/14651858.CD013574.

8. Andrist E, Clarke RG, Harding M. Paved with good intentions: hospital visitation restrictions in the age of coronavirus disease 2019. *Pediatr Crit Care Med.* 2020. https://doi.org/10.1097/PCC.0000000000002506. Epub ahead of print. PMID: 32541371; PMCID: PMC7314338.

9. Ferguson NM, Laydon D, Nedjati-Gilani G, Imai N, Ainslie K, Baguelin M, et al. Report 9: Impact of non-pharmaceutical interventions (NPIs) to reduce COVID-19 mortality and healthcare demand. https://www.imperial.ac.uk/media/imperial-college/medicine/mrc-gida/2020-03-16-COVID19-Report-9.pdf Accessed 6 July 2020.

10. Lebow JL. Family in the age of COVID-19. *Fam Process.* 2020;59(2):309–312. https://doi.org/10.1111/famp.12543.

11. Needham DM, Davidson J, Cohen H, et al. Improving long-term outcomes after discharge from intensive care unit: report from a stakeholders' conference. *Crit Care Med.* 2012;40:502–509.

12. Schmidt M, Azoulay E. Having a loved one in the ICU: the forgotten family. *Curr Opin Crit Care.* 2012;18:540–547.

13. Pochard F, Darmon M, Fassier T, et al. French FAMIREA study group: symptoms of anxiety and depression in family members of intensive care unit patients before discharge or death. A prospective multi-center study. *J Crit Care.* 2005;20:90–96.

14. Pochard F, Azoulay E, Chevret S, et al. French FAMIREA Group: symptoms of anxiety and depression in family members of intensive care unit patients: ethical hypothesis regarding decision-making capacity. *Crit Care Med.* 2001;29:1893–1897.

15. Lautrette A, Darmon M, Megarbane B, et al. A communication strategy and brochure for relatives of patients dying in the ICU. *N Engl J Med.* 2007;356:469–478.

16. Kentish-Barnes N, Chaize M, Seegers V, et al. Complicated grief after death of a relative in the intensive care unit. *Eur Respir J.* 2015;45:1341–1352.

17. Cameron JI, Chu LM, Matte A, Tomlinson G, Chan L, Thomas C. RECOVER program investigators (phase 1: towards RECOVER); Canadian critical care trials group. One-year outcomes in care- givers of critically ill patients. *N Engl J Med.* 2016; 374:1831–1841.

18. Van Beusekom I, Bakhshi-Raiez F, de Keizer NF, Dongelmans DA, van der Schaaf M. Reported burden on informal care- givers of ICU survivors: a literature review. *Crit Care.* 2016;20:16–21.

19. Torres J, Carvalho D, Molinos E, et al. The impact of the patient's post intensive care syndrome components on caregiver's burden. *Med Int.* 2017;41:454–460 [article in English, Spanish].

20. Brown SM, Rozenblum R, Aboumatar H, et al. Defining patient and family engagement in the intensive care unit. *Am J Respir Crit Care Med.* 2015;191(3):358–360.

21. Verhaeghe S, Defloor T, Van Zuuren F, Duijnstee M, Grypdonck M. The needs and experiences of family members of adult patients in an intensive care unit: a review of the literature. *J Clin Nurs.* 2005;14(4):501–509. https://doi.org/10.1111/j.1365-2702.2004.01081.x. 15807758.

22. Molter NC. Families are not visitors in the critical care unit. *Dimens Crit Care Nurs.* 1994;13:2–3.

23. Davidson JE, Aslakson RA, Long AC, et al. Guidelines for family-centered Care in the neonatal, pediatric, and adult ICU. *Crit Care Med.* 2017;45(1):103–128.

24. Ely EW. The ABCDEF bundle: science and philosophy of how ICU liberation serves patients and families. *Crit Care Med.* 2017;45:321–330.

25. Pun BT, Balas MC, Barnes-Daly MA, et al. Caring for critically ill patients with the ABCDEF bundle: results of the ICU liberation collaborative in over 15,000 adults. *Crit Care Med.* 2019;47(1):3–14.

26. Bjoern Z, Camenisch SA, Schefold JC. *Interventions in post-intensive care syndrome-family, critical care medicine*; 2020. https://doi.org/10.1097/CCM.0000000000004450. June 25, 2020 - Volume Online First - Issue.

27. Carson SS, Cox CE, Wallenstein S, et al. Effect of palliative care-led meetings for families of patients with chronic critical illness: a randomized clinical trial. *JAMA.* 2016;316: 51–62.

28. Kentish-Barnes N, Chevret S, Champigneulle B, et al. Famirea study group: effect of a condolence letter on grief symptoms among relatives of patients who died in the ICU: a randomized clinical trial. *Intensive Care Med.* 2017;43:473–484.

29. Heras La Calle G, Oviés ÁA, Tello VG. A plan for improving the humanization of intensive care units. *Intensive Care Med.* 2017;43(4):547–549.

30. Heras La Calle G. *My Favorite Slide: The ICU and the Human Care Bundle.* NEJM Catalyst; 2018. April 5.

31. Nin Vaeza N, Martin Delgado MC, Heras La Calle G. Humanizing intensive care: toward a human-centered care ICU model. *Crit Care Med.* 2020;48(3):385–390.

32. Newyorktime. https://www.nytimes.com/2020/03/29/health/coronavirus-hospital-visit-ban.html. Accessed 6 July 2020.

33. Shojaei A, Salari P. *COVID-19 and off label use of drugs: an ethical viewpoint.* Daru; 2020:1–5. https://doi.org/10.1007/s40199-020-00351-y. May 8. Epub ahead of print. PMID: 32385829; PMCID: PMC7207985.

34. Wakam GK, Montgomery JR, Biesterveld BE, Brown CS. Not dying alone - modern compassionate Care in the Covid-19 pandemic. *N Engl J Med.* 2020;382(24). https://doi.org/10.1056/NEJMp2007781, e88 [Epub 2020 Apr 14].

35. Gries CJ, Engelberg RA, Kross EK, et al. Predictors of symptoms of post-traumatic stress and depression in family members after patient death in the ICU. *Chest.* 2010;137(2): 280–287.

36. Phua J, Weng L, Ling L, et al. Intensive care management of coronavirus disease 2019 (COVID-19): challenges and recommendations. *Lancet Respir Med.* 2020. https://doi.org/10.1016/S2213-2600(20)30161-2. published online April 6.

37. Berwick DM, Kotagal M. Restricted visiting hours in ICUs: time to change. *JAMA.* 2004;292:736–737.

38. Lai J, Ma S, Wang Y, et al. Factors associated with mental health outcomes among health care workers exposed to coronavirus disease 2019. *JAMA Netw Open.* 2020;3(3). https://doi.org/10.1001/jamanetworkopen.2020.3976, e203976.

39. Lewnard JA, Lo NC. Scientific and ethical basis for social-distancing interventions against COVID-19. *Lancet Infect Dis.* 2020. https://doi.org/10.1016/S1473-3099(20)30190-0.

40. Rogers S. Why can't I visit? The ethics of visitation restrictions—lessons learned from SARS. *Crit Care.* 2004;8:300–302.

41. Declaración del comité de bioética de España sobre el derecho y deber de facilitar el acompañamiento y la asistencia espiritual a los pacientes con covid-19 al final de sus

vidas y en situaciones de especial vulnerabilidad. n.d. http://assets.comitedebioetica.es/files/documentacion/CBE_Declaracion_sobre_acompanamiento_COVID19.pdf.

42. Hart JL, Turnbull AE, Oppenheim IM, Courtright KR. Family-centered care during the COVID-19 era. *J Pain Symptom Manag.* 2020. https://doi.org/10.1016/j.jpainsymman.2020.04.017. S0885-3924(20)30208-6. Epub ahead of print. PMID: 32333961; PMCID: PMC7175858.

43. Azoulay E, Kentish-Barnes N. A 5-point strategy for improved connection with relatives of critically ill patients with COVID-19. *Lancet Respir Med.* 2020;8(6). https://doi.org/10.1016/S2213-2600(20)30223-X, e52.

44. Jabre P, Tazarourte AE. Offering the opportunity for family to be present during cardiopulmonary resuscitation: 1-year assessment. *Intensive Care Med.* 2014;40:981–987.

45. Beesley SJ, Hopkins RO, Francis L, et al. Let them in: family presence during intensive care unit procedures. *Ann Am Thorac Soc.* 2016;13(7):1155–1159. https://doi.org/10.1513/AnnalsATS.201511-754OI. 27104301.

46. Lederman Z. Family presence during cardiopulmonary resuscitation in the Covid-19 era. *Resuscitation.* 2020;151:137–138. https://doi.org/10.1016/j.resuscitation.2020.04.028.

47. Robert R, Kentish-Barnes N, Boyer A, Laurent A, Azoulay E, Reignier J. Ethical dilemmas due to the Covid-19 pandemic. Version 2. *Ann Intensive Care.* 2020;10(1):84. https://doi.org/10.1186/s13613-020-00702-7. PMID: 32556826; PMCID: PMC7298921.

48. Nelson JE, Puntillo KA, Pronovost PJ, et al. In their own words: patients and families define high-quality palliative care in the intensive care unit. *Crit Care Med.* 2010;38(3):808–818.

49. Azoulay E, Pochard F, Kentish-Barnes N, et al. Risk of post-traumatic stress symptoms in family members of intensive care unit patients. *Am J Respir Crit Care Med.* 2005;171(9):987–994.

50. https://semicyuc.org/pacientes/ Accessed 6 July 2020.

51. nopanicovid.com Accessed 6 July 2020.

52. Curtis JR, Kross EK, Stapleton RD. The importance of addressing advance care planning and decisions about do-not-resuscitate orders during novel coronavirus 2019 (COVID-19). *JAMA.* 2020;323:1771–1772.

53. Estella Á. Compassionate communication and end-of-life Care for Critically ill Patients with SARS-CoV-2 infection. *J Clin Ethics.* 2020;31(2):191–193. 32585665.

54. Montauk TR, Kuhl EA. COVID-related family separation and trauma in the intensive care unit. *Psychol Trauma Theory Res Pract Policy.* 2020. https://doi.org/10.1037/tra0000839. Advance online publication.

55. Wallace CL, Wladkowski SP, Gibson A, White P. Grief during the COVID-19 pandemic: considerations for palliative care providers. *J Pain Symptom Manag.* 2020;60(1):e70–e76. https://doi.org/10.1016/j.jpainsymman.2020.04.012.

COVID-19: A health-care worker's perspective

5

Rishi Suresh[a], Ryan J. Logue[b], Deepa B. Gotur[b,c], and Steven H. Hsu[b,c]
[a]*Texas A&M School of Medicine, College Station, TX, United States,* [b]*Department of Medicine, Houston Methodist Hospital, Houston, TX, United States,* [c]*Weill Cornell Medicine, New York, NY, United States*

Introduction

The coronavirus disease 2019 (COVID-19) pandemic took the world by surprise in 2020, rapidly overwhelming our societies, economies, and health-care systems. The health-care workers (HCWs), hospital administrators, government leaders, and public health officials all rushed to coordinate the response in order to contain its global spread. Early on, it became clear that the virus was highly contagious and had a longer latent (yet transmissible) period when compared with previous pandemics. During the early dynamics in Wuhan, China, the basic reproductive number (R_0) was 2.2–2.7, suggesting a doubling time of number of infected persons of 6–7 days.[1] The spread of the disease has been further exacerbated by limitations in testing and medical supplies, disconcerting guidelines, conflicting media information, and whether policies are instituted and enforced to attempt to "flatten the curve" as well as the timeliness of health-related political efforts. At the same time, a swarming number of fast-track publications and interventions overwhelmed frontline HCWs with excessive and misrepresented study conclusions that needed to be implemented at the bedside. Some high-profile publications were even retracted limiting further therapeutic options. Facing these uncertainties, HCWs have been battling with immense physical and psychological stress from a surge of clinical work, staff shortage, bed crunch, potential lack of personal protective equipment (PPE) and drugs, and profound ethical conflicts. Above all, HCWs grapple with the risks that the exposure to the virus could have not only for themselves but for their families. By June 2020, The International Council of Nursing reported an estimate of 230,000 infected HCWs and over 600 nurses died based on information collected on 30 countries from national nursing associations, government figures, and media reports.[2] In this chapter, we explore the multitude of challenges confronting the frontline providers during this COVID-19 pandemic.

Legal and ethical dilemmas
Resource scarcity

The COVID-19 crisis and the shortage of resources have generated a multitude of ethically challenging scenarios. Fundamentally, there is a clash between utilitarian and deontological principles in the way that the health-care system approaches the distribution of COVID-related resources. Prior to COVID-19, HCWs treated individuals using a deontological framework. According to that principle, each patient is treated as an individual, and the decision to provide a lifesaving intervention is made exclusively on the individuals and their conditions.[3] The current crisis has necessitated a more utilitarian framework, where the focus is on maximizing saved lives or therapeutic outcomes for the greatest number of people. This means that some individuals would likely not receive potentially lifesaving interventions because of their underlying comorbidities, in favor of utilizing these resources for patients with a higher likelihood of success.[4]

In Italy and Spain, providers were forced to make excruciating decisions regarding resource access to patients based on factors such as comorbidities and severity of respiratory failure. The Italian Society of Anesthesia, Analgesia, Resuscitation and Intensive Care (SIAARTI) of the ethics section described the possible need for a utilitarian approach in which factors like age could be utilized along with comorbidities and functional status to create intensive care unit (ICU) admission criteria.[5] In fact, the SIAARTI guidelines described that each admission to the ICU should be considered a "trial" in which patients are reassessed on a daily basis to determine whether the use of scarce lifesaving resources such as ventilators are properly allocated. Such situations were exceptionally challenging to witness for frontline HCWs who previously had operated using a framework that offered access to all individuals.[6]

A significant amount of attention in the early days of the pandemic was focused on the need for ventilators; however, resource scarcity created moral-ethical problems that went beyond ventilator access. Several investigational drugs that were potentially effective in treating COVID-19 [such as hydroxychloroquine (HCQ), remdesivir, lopinavir-ritonavir, or convalescent plasma] have a limited availability, and sometimes have required the adventure of strict institutional policies to restrict their use to a preselected population.

The scarcity of PPE has also forced HCWs to rethink several aspects of medical management. For example, when a patient requires resuscitation, there is an immediate moral conflict between the importance of early intervention and the need to properly protect oneself prior to entering a COVID-19-positive patient's room. The amount of time taken to don PPE prior to entering a patient's room can delay the effectiveness of the resuscitation efforts.[3] Specifically, chest compression generates aerosols if the patient is not already intubated. Therefore prior to attempting resuscitation, it is imperative that the HCW appropriately protect themselves. And then, the prevalence of the disease in some areas has made that in many instances, all patients should be treated as suspected cases thus limiting the celerity or even availability of certain treatments for the entire population.

Directing a health-care team on cardiopulmonary resuscitation (CPR) efforts to restore spontaneous circulation and breathing of a patient certainly utilizes a significant amount of PPE. HCWs have searched for ways to streamline this process to ensure that patient's wishes are followed while proper PPE is conserved. Discussions regarding advance directives and do-not-resuscitate (DNR) status are initiated early on in a patient's hospital course. Identifying those who would not want CPR and those who would benefit from CPR can guide in formulating treatment plans and limits. Routine discussions regarding goals of care and code status with patients and their families should be part of the standard practices when treating hospitalized patients with COVID-19, particularly in high-risk patients. Other strategies to ensure safety include having extra PPE in emergency carts, limiting the number of essential staff, using an external mechanical chest compressor and protective barriers over the patient to minimize aerosolization, and using airway intubation by dedicated or most experienced staff.[7]

The issue of conducting CPR in the context of the COVID-19 pandemic has sparked ongoing debate with viewpoints such as DNR for all COVID-19 patients.[3] A professional society like the Belgian Resuscitation Council recommends avoiding CPR when providers' safety is not met and in those with little chance of good functional outcome.[7] Similarly for patients recovering yet requiring long-term ventilation, conflicting recommendations exist on performing tracheostomy. While it can expedite weaning and freeing up an ICU bed, it is also aerosol-generating, requiring enhanced PPE measures. Even outside of the COVID-19 context, there are differences in the timing of tracheostomy. This pandemic has added another uncertainty on the timing of it, (if at all offered) due to sustained positivity of the virological testing.[8] Again, these approaches represent a utilitarian mindset to maximize PPE resource utilization while achieving a standard of safety.

Clearly, the ethical and moral circumstances involved in resource allocation are complex. In order for these principles to be applied in a consistent manner, professional societies, institutions, states, and national governing bodies should create guidelines that discuss best practices for managing these complex situations. Furthermore, it would be beneficial to have local ethics committees to assist in making difficult decisions about complicated ethical cases and to ease the burden of HCWs from having to navigate these ethical issues by themselves.

Managing the workforce

The pervasiveness of COVID-19 creates tremendous concern that HCWs of all specialties are likely to be at risk of exposure at work. Various questions have been raised regarding the responsibility in treating potentially COVID-positive patients, especially when doing so places the providers and their families at risk. The American Medical Association Code of Ethics describes the physician's duty to treat, which states: "Because of their commitment to care for the sick and injured, individual physicians have an obligation to provide urgent medical care during disasters. This ethical obligation holds even in the face of greater than usual risks to their own safety, health, or life."[9] The code of ethics suggests that it would not necessarily be permissible to excuse oneself from the duties of patient care due to increased personal risk. This generates a sense of *prima facie* obligation to serve, which the frontline HCWs of Wuhan, Italy, New York, and essentially all over the world, did not shy away from when facing the first wave. During the initial phase of pandemic, China summoned the workforce and resources at a national level to support Wuhan, while Italy and the United States recruited volunteers and traveling staff to the major disease epicenters and even graduated trainees ahead of time to join the workforce.[10] Major international medical societies like the Society of Critical Care Medicine reached out to their members and were able to recruit and organize volunteer critical care clinicians to respond to places like New York.[11] Some areas also recruited retired providers to aid with the epidemic.[12] Most of the recruits had different backgrounds and specialties. However, the increased demand for HCWs on the front lines was quickly met by a relative shortage of PPE. Such situations placed HCWs with the dilemma to stand up to the challenge posed by the pandemic, while being concerned for their own safety due to lack of PPE and shortcoming of basic safety.

A significant amount of the workforce falls into the groups considered to be at risk of COVID-19. Approximately 22% of nurses and 29% of physicians in the United States are over the age of 55, placing them at increased risk of severe disease.[13] Furthermore, those with comorbidities such as hypertension, diabetes, obesity, asthma, and immunocompromised states are at even higher risk.[14,15] HCWs that have either at-risk or high-risk individuals at home are also faced with difficult choices of the possibility of bringing home the virus. Hospitals have addressed this challenge in various ways. Some at-risk staff were asked to minimize contact with patients on the front lines.[16] Others have opted for more individualized approaches, in which HCWs are provided choices regarding whether they would like to stay and treat patients or relocate to another service for less exposure.[15]

The decision to remove oneself from the clinical environment is challenging. Some HCWs have detailed the conflict between the need for themselves and their family to be protected, while serving their obligation to their patients.[17] HCWs that remove themselves from the clinical environment do so feeling slightly uncomfortable or guilty, and even potential perceived bias from others.[18,19] Even if HCWs recuse themselves from the front line, there are several ways in which they are able to add significant value in the health-care setting. The accelerated shift toward telehealth during the pandemic has allowed for physicians to actively treat patients even during this crisis. Furthermore, some hospitals have allowed some interventional specialties to take call, but not actively round on inpatient units where patients could be COVID-19 positive.[16] Finally, elderly HCWs have a wealth of experience and knowledge, and they are able to provide additional support to their younger colleagues and trainees during this time, including academic conferences and clinical guidance.

While some hospitals have opted to protect those that are at the highest risk of having complications related to COVID-19, others have cautioned against intentionally placing low-risk individuals in high-risk situations. After all, the disease still carries a significant risk of serious complications in younger low-risk patient population. Managing the workforce in the face of these ethical considerations is challenging and is likely to evolve as the pandemic progresses.

Am I protected?
PPE availability

As COVID-19 exponentially surged in the United States, there were several concerns regarding the availability of proper PPE. During the initial phase of the pandemic, hospital workers were frustrated by the lack of access to PPE, and guidelines regarding its use seemed to be constantly changing. An early estimate in China suggested that infection of HCWs was as high as 29%.[20] This percentage dramatically decreased as hospitals refined their protocols for PPE use. Tragically, HCWs are not spared from succumbing to the disease.[21] By July 2020, the Centers for Disease Control and Prevention (CDC) reported over 90,000 cases of COVID-19 infection in HCWs and at least 500 deaths in the United States.[22]

Initially, some hospitals were forced to come up with emergency solutions to provide necessary PPE, from relying on community donations to working with organizations and even to provide three-dimensional printed face shields. The shortage of N95 respirators has forced HCWs to reuse them following decontamination or after a certain waiting period beyond the manufacturer's recommendation. Several volunteer groups were created throughout the United States that focused on collecting community resources to provide hospitals with appropriate PPE. Since the start of the pandemic, hospitals have become more efficient with their PPE use, and the CDC guidelines have been refined to allow for reuse of PPE in multiple settings. Nevertheless, the availability of PPE will likely remain a consistent problem throughout the course of the pandemic.[23,24]

The continually changing CDC guidelines with respect to PPE usage were often a cause for stress and anxiety among providers on the front line, as the recommendations appeared to be constrained by PPE availability rather than by evidence-based practices. For example, at one point during the pandemic, CDC guidelines encouraged HCWs to wear bandanas to protect themselves when masks were not available.[25] In the initial phase of the pandemic and with shortages of masks, CDC also did not recommend the general public to use face masks in an effort to prevent diverting them from health-care facilities. This strategy could have worsened the epidemiological spread. Face masks have also confronted political innuendos which might have some influence in the spread of the disease. In addition, epidemiologic surges and increasing hospital admissions have propelled the enhanced need for more resources, creating in some cases chaotic scenarios that prompted media and general public attention.

In an effort to conserve PPE, hospitals have implemented innovative solutions for the routine care of patients. In the ICU, getting chest X-rays without having the machine enter the room, placing intravenous pumps outside the rooms, nonstandard setting hemodialysis, and distant ventilator monitors are feasible and used strategies that have minimized the times that providers spend inside the patient's room minimizing not only the time of exposure but also, through limiting the number of entries, reducing the use of the scarce PPE's.[24] Additional measures include reserving the highest levels of PPE, such as N95 or powered air-purifying respirator, for the management of COVID-19 patients and aerosol-generating or lengthy procedures.

Protecting HCWs at work and home

Several studies have demonstrated that COVID-19 can easily contaminate various surfaces inside the hospital.[26,27] Areas like break rooms and nursing stations, shared computers, and communal phones are particularly susceptible. Thus cleaning of surfaces is required to avoid cross contamination. A recent CDC study found that the shoes that providers wear in the hospital have the potential to carry the virus and serve as possible modes of transmission into the HCW's home as well.[28] Therefore attention needs to be directed to the movements within the working environment and to and from home, observing that personal gears and belongings need to be cleaned thoroughly and treated with caution.

Caring for patients outside the identified areas deserves a special mention. As HCWs are typically moved to wear sufficient PPE when caring for a COVID-19 patient, this may be laxed if the patient presents no clear diagnosis or rather is admitted with a non-related condition. This portends the danger of transmission as the pandemic progresses and the prevalence becomes increased. Patients could be positive and spreading infection although admitted with other conditions and sometimes the delay in identifying them, whether is because of waiting for a routine test or simply because of the lack of suspicion, endangers the HCW if nonadequate protection is embraced. This might be even more complicated while some institutions might be limiting the use of some PPEs to predetermined areas. Under these conditions, determining whether a patient is positive is imperative to initiate appropriate isolation and to protect staff and other patients. However, testing continues to be an issue in many countries, especially in areas where community outbreaks lead to excessive surge demand. Furthermore, the imperfect sensitivity of approximately 70% in SARS-CoV-2 polymerase chain reaction testing determines a significant number of false negatives. In regions with high number of cases and positive rates, HCWs should exercise standard precautions and assume all patients are COVID-19 in order to appropriately protect and reduce the risk of exposure.[29,30]

Mental and psychological well-being of HCWs

While COVID-19 presents a real threat of serious physical illness, there is also a significant threat to the mental and psychological well-being of the providers. In previous influenza outbreaks in China, staff absenteeism was a significant issue.[31] Various factors contributed to the shortage and loss of productivity, including numerous absentees with reported upper respiratory tract symptoms, fear of occupational hazard, and having caregiving duties at home due to the closing of school and child-care facilities. Workforce preparation and planning during patient surges, staff shortages must be taken into consideration. To account for these deficits, hospitals have hired traveling staff in the United States, redistributed internal workforces, and closely monitored symptomatic staff with explicit guidelines for postexposure testing and return to work policies.

The constant stress of treating COVID-19 patients among ever-changing guidelines, handling significantly more patients than normal, working in suboptimal makeshift settings, and with inadequate PPE, all contribute to overwhelm HCWs and have tangible impacts on their mental health and well-being.[32] During this pandemic, HCWs are often required to take more roles including the one handling end-of-life issues in an environment that has proven to be very hostile for patients and families. In an effort to minimize the spread of the virus, hospitals have created limitations on the number of visitors, time allowed for those visits, and most institutions have implemented a no-visitor policy for ICU patients. Thus HCWs engage thoroughly in end-of-life care discussions without the benefit of face-to-face visits. Furthermore, they are called upon to provide comfort and support in the immediate days and hours leading up to a patient's death. Providers have adapted to these challenges by involving palliative care services early on in hospitalizations to ease the transition toward end-of-life care.[24]

On a personal level, the pandemic has brought a sense of social isolation as HCWs often distance themselves from their family members for fear of infecting them. Prior to the pandemic, burnout and moral injury were already quite high among HCWs in areas such as the emergency room and ICU. The intense nature of the pandemic amplifies these issues. Hospitals must be proactive in protecting HCWs from the moral and psychological injury that comes with being in these difficult environments.

Institutions have attempted to confront these issues in several different ways. For example, during the initial Wuhan outbreak, the delegated medical teams often incorporated psychologists to help support the staff. Most institutions have provided similar strategies and services to help their staff to cope with the stress, and the CDC has made resources available as well.[33] Furthermore, hosting regular town halls, or providing access to mindfulness sessions or telehealth counseling visits, having a dedicated staff center and hotlines for emotional support by psychologists and social workers are proposed to ensure that HCWs receive the help they need.[33]

What if I get sick?

Despite the proper use of PPE, HCWs are not fully exempt from exposure to COVID-19 and get sick. As nearly a quarter million HCWs are infected by COVID-19 globally has been reported as of June 2020, institutions must plan ahead for those recovered to resume duty.[2] Most return-to-work policies have focused on either symptom- or testing-based strategies. For instance, CDC recommends a symptom-based strategy, providers are excluded from working either until after 10 days since the first symptoms appeared or until 3 days have passed since recovery. In a test-based strategy, health-care providers are excluded from work until their symptoms resolve, and they receive negative results from two consecutive respiratory specimens.[34]

In these situations, concerns raise not only for the individual health of the provider but also with regard to potentially exposing their family members. While trying to recover from the disease, providers may have to find alternate accommodations or means of self-isolation to avoid such risk. In many countries including the United States, hotels and local college dormitories have attempted to provide accommodations to health-care providers helping with the COVID-19 crisis.[35–39] Similarly, hospitals in Italy and China provided meals and lodging to frontline HCWs to allow them to ensure proper social distancing.[40] One specific hospital in Italy utilized a hotel and set up a system complete with "dirty paths" (where HCWs could travel), regular temperature, and symptom screening to quickly identify potentially infected individuals.[40] While these accommodations provide HCWs with the ability to relocate while they are potentially able to transmit the virus, they still face significant challenges in taking care of their responsibilities outside of the hospital. An equally important matter is the possible exposure of the HCW in the "outside" environment and the possibility of bringing the infection to the inside. This has been a common in most areas of the United States where the rate of HCW infection has been similar to the general population in the area.

How to treat the unknown?

Since the beginning of the pandemic, the amount of research and information regarding best practices for the treatment has flooded publications and media. Amidst this deluge of information, it has been challenging for providers to stay up-to-date with their management strategies and care of patients. As of July 1, 2020, there were 27,778 publications indexed in the LitCovid website.[41] Further complicating the problem is that studies on the effectiveness of a particular drug can often conflict, leaving the provider unsure of whether it is likely to provide a benefit to the patient. Sometimes, high-profile studies have been ultimately retracted, leading to further confusion.

In the vast majority of clinical situations, there are thorough guidelines for management. However, in this pandemic, the guidelines for treatment are changing constantly based on data that appear at a rapid pace. Noise has been generated by intrinsic factors of the different studies such the number of subjects included, the methodology of the study, and the lack of randomization among others. Some institution studies chose to forgo the use of control groups called by the need for treatment making it difficult to stablish real comparable data. In addition, there is hunger and urgency for the consecution of treatment options, and any study has immediate attention in the media.[42]

Many experimental drugs, some of them new and some old but redirected, have appeared as treatment alternatives. HCWs must consider whether it is appropriate to treat the COVID-19 patients with the experimental drug outside the context of a research protocol. The code of ethics of the physician-patient relationship and those of the investigator-subject relationship may not be aligned. This is a challenging path for physicians in large academic centers who are fulfilling both roles of a researcher and a clinician. Physicians have a fiduciary duty to act in the patient's best interest and recommend treatments to patients based on their clinical judgment, as long as the treatment is within a reasonable standard of care. Research occurs outside the context of a beneficence-based relationship with a goal of acquisition of generalizable knowledge and, for most research, there is not a clear expectation of benefit for the patient. In a situation where a clinician is facing a patient with life-threatening progression of the disease, the three ethical principles of nonmaleficence, informed consent, and benevolence comes into play. Keeping with the patient's best interest and on the premises of helping the dying patient, a consenting patient should be provided with treatment that may still be unproven in research studies. The classic example is that of an old drug that treats Ebola, remdesivir which was repurposed to use in the SARS-CoV-2 pandemic and was given emergency use authorization. In academic medical centers, patients often have access to several trials that are seeking to improve outcomes and patient care. In such settings, providers are more likely to be kept up to date with the available therapies that researchers are trying to use. However, community hospitals might struggle to access some of these specialized therapies, limiting their ability to optimally care for their patients. Nevertheless, as the pandemic progresses, access to certain drugs such as HCQ (initially considered to be effective) or remdesivir has been limited, forcing difficult decisions on who qualifies to receive the limited doses that exist.

Commitment of the HCW on education of the trainees

The training of medical students, nursing, and allied health professionals was substantially impacted in the United States as a result of COVID-19. Students and trainees were at first not allowed to take care of COVID-19 patients, due to concerns regarding PPE shortage. In March, the American Association of Medical Colleges and the Liaison Committee on Medical Education published a recommendation advising that students be pulled from clinical environments for a few weeks while schools identified alternative learning plans.[43] Students were placed in alternative learning environments, including online learning modules, taking part in didactics, or even seeing patients through telehealth encounters. The decision to restrict trainees from seeing COVID-positive patients is often based on a desire to preserve PPE and to prevent exposure. However, others argue that not allowing students to treat COVID-positive patients deprives them of the learning experience gained from being actively involved in a pandemic. Nevertheless, some schools are finding ways to involve their trainees by assisting with outpatient clinics, with telehealth visits, or helping with inpatients that are not COVID positive.[43] Some have even come up with more novel uses for medical students, such as training them to supplement respiratory therapists.[44] Finally, even if medical students are not actively involved in treating COVID-positive patients, HCWs can still teach trainees about these patients through patient rounds or in case conferences.

On the contrary, students in the last year of school in hard-hit areas such as New York or Massachusetts were provided the opportunity to graduate early and join the physician workforce.[45] The decisions on whether to allow students to pursue these opportunities were often made on a school-by-school basis and required a state-level involvement in order to provide the appropriate licensure. Countries like Italy passed the Cura Italia decree, which allowed all medical schools in the country to advance their students into the workforce at a much faster rate.[46] Similarly, a UK-wide approach was used to allow British medical students to join the National Health Service earlier than previously would have been possible.[47]

COVID-19 has also profoundly affected residency education. Regularly scheduled didactics and educational opportunities have been disrupted as a result of clinical duties overwhelming senior staff.[48] Initially, the guidance from the Accreditation Council for Graduate Medical Education was for residents to avoid treating COVID-19 patients altogether.[49] However, this was quickly amended to allow residents to see COVID patients, given that they had appropriate training in management and personal protection. Residents working in epicenters often have to support in the field and found themselves fearing the same issues that other HCWs face—such as concerns regarding PPE accessibility and protecting their loved ones—in addition to other issues specific to their role as trainees. For example, they also have to worry about duty hour regulations, patient caps, or the impact of quarantine periods on their eventual graduation. As the pandemic evolves, institutions are finding ways to incorporate the workforce with proper protection and education on how to treat COVID-19.[49]

Physicians as innovators and researchers

This pandemic has given an opportunity to the rapid adaption of innovative solutions to the clinical problems faced at the bedside. For example, HCWs were involved in inventing makeshift ventilators, aerosol containing boxes for use during intubations, or even attempting to use artificial intelligence to diagnose COVID-19 from a computed tomography scan.[50–52] As the pandemic progressed, there was a rapid shift toward telehealth visits for routine clinical care. These visits also were useful in limiting provider exposure and further communal spread. HCWs throughout the world have embraced their roles as researchers, developing trials that evaluate potential vaccines, repurposing previously used drugs, and developing ideas for novel therapies such as convalescent plasma.

The influence (or "mis-influence") of social media

As the "infodemic" created a cloudy consensus as to best practice management algorithms, HCWs were also challenged with the profound influence of social media on patients and families. The various social media platforms, with billions of viewers daily, have the potential to either support or hamper public health efforts. It is estimated that during lockdown, social media traffic was up 61% overall and instant messaging features attracting 50% greater usage than usual.[53] According to a leading social media management company, from March to April 2020, health-care posts increased by 5.3% and conventional media outlet posts increased by 8.9%.[54] With an increase in both social media content and consumer traffic, opinions, viewpoints, and at times misleading information flooded and created sometimes an uneasy environment for the HCW. As an example, a study published in the "British Medical Journal" during the same time period found that 25% of the top 75 viewed COVID-19-related videos on YouTube contained grossly misleading information that was being disseminated to millions of viewers worldwide.[55] In light of such findings, prominent social media platforms have introduced fact-checking protocols for obvious misinformation related to the pandemic.

Despite this, it has been shown that people seek and share content based on preconceived perceptions. For instance, Dr. Rasmus Nielsen, Oxford professor and director at Reuters, found that in numerous developed countries, people who politically leaned left trusted the media more than the government, whereas those who leaned right trusted the government more than the media.[56] In addition to inaccurate, misleading, and conflicting information, social media can also affect the psyche of the viewers. Evidence shows that during the lockdown, using social media to gain information about COVID-19 has led to considerable spread of anxiety related to the pandemic.[57]

From the perspective of the HCWs, such a profound dissent among available social media content made it more challenging to be a community leader and educator during the pandemic. While HCWs have been vigilant to scrutinize blatantly incorrect claims, other controversial posts have made it challenging for HCWs to take a stand. Perhaps, the most infamous example of bridging the "infodemic" with social media and politics is that of U.S. President Donald Trump and his early endorsement of an antimalarial medication as a potential COVID-19 treatment. On March 19 and 21, he tweeted messages in favor of immediate approval for HCQ, citing a recent French study that indicated HCQ with azithromycin led to significantly decreased COVID-19 viral loads.[58] However, after various critiques of the study and withdrawal of its trial by WHO, Trump's top public health advisors including Drs. Anthony Fauci and Rick Bright have declared the message as dangerous. Another example is the declarations of the presidential candidate Joe Biden against the travel ban declared by the U.S. government in January 2020. Usage of media by candidate and diverting the attention from health to political arena was later retracted, in April, by his own campaign.

Divergent views on health policy

Response to the SARS-CoV-2 pandemic has varied across the globe, with health policy ranging from stringent lockdown to attempts at achieving herd immunity. Nevertheless, there were challenging sociopolitical and economic decisions made to optimize health-care management, political response, and financial policy.

Being the epicenter of the viral outbreak, the Chinese government officials were criticized for controlling and censorship of information at the expense of public safety. As early as December 31, 2019, Western outlets such as "The New York Times" were reporting on a possible novel viral outbreak, while Chinese citizens were largely unaware.[59] Doctors including Li Wenliang warned of a novel virus similar to SARS. After he sent a text message warning his colleagues to wear appropriate PPE, he was called to the Chinese Public Security Bureau to discuss his concerns. He later succumbed to complications from the SARS-CoV-2 virus.

As the virus spread out of China during the initial phases of the pandemic, neighboring East Asian countries were forced to act swiftly to mitigate the spread of the pandemic. Notably, Taiwan (seven deaths as of late June 2020) quickly closed its borders, halted the export of surgical masks, and the government implemented contract tracing and mobile SIM tracking to identify that those relegated to quarantine were actually following the rules. Health officials in Taiwan held public briefing sessions daily and implemented that businesses screen entrance with temperature monitoring and require customers to use hand sanitizer prior to access.[60]

By the time the virus had reached Europe, there was little time for advanced planning to contain the virus. In the short span from February 21 to March 22, 2020, Italy went from identifying the first case of COVID-19 to complete shutdown of the country. Early on, the Italian officials recognized that they were unable to deliver population-centric care. Emergency declarations were met with skepticism. This was not unique to Italy, as an alarming degree of similar mindset spread through Europe and North America. As the general public and policymakers dabbled in partial policy solutions, the virus spread at alarming rates. Ultimately, the Italian missteps in the early phases of the pandemic helped the rest of the world to understand two major key factors to mitigating viral spread. As quoted by the head of the Italian Protezione Civile, "the virus moves faster than bureaucracy," underscoring the essence of time. Secondly, the number of resources, both human and economic, required to beat the virus requires a war-like mobilization.[61]

In the United States, the earliest wave of the SARS-CoV-2 pandemic was reported in Washington state, followed shortly after with devastatingly high rates of infection in New York state. On March 10, 2020, New York governor Andrew Cuomo established the nation's first coronavirus containment zone in New Rochelle, followed 6 days later by a tri-state coalition between New York, New Jersey, and Connecticut that formulated the rules of a shutdown. In the subsequent weeks, cases eventually amassed 370,000 with the official death toll over 23,000 people.[62] Further responses from individual state governors and the federal government have been controversial to date. The pandemic has left policymakers at odds in regard to the responsibility of the public health response, as state governors have adapted individualized plans regarding closing, "lockdown," and reopening. The federal response included President Donald Trump signing bill H.R. 6074 to support national efforts to combat the virus, as well as The Families First Coronavirus Response Act. The latter bill required private health-care plans to provide coverage for COVID-19 testing and visits, paid sick leave for COVID-19, funding for women, infants, and children, as well as increased funding for Medicaid. Finally, federal government agencies such as the CDC and the United States Department of Labor have outlined extensive recommendations regarding recommendations for PPE and safe work practices.

Finally, some countries have adopted a more *"laissez-faire"* approach to containing the SARS-CoV-2 outbreak. Namely, Sweden has opted for minimal restrictions and advocated for personal responsibility. This approach led many to hope that the country would reach herd immunity as quickly as possible. As of May 2020, Sweden's rate of daily new cases and cumulative deaths per million have outpaced other Scandinavian countries threefold.[63] To date, Swedish hospitals have managed the onslaught of COVID-19 patients. As countries around the world look to reopen and stimulate economic growth during the pandemic, some have looked to Sweden as an exemplary model. The World Health Organization's (WHO) top experts have pointed to Sweden's social responsibility model as an ideal model as countries begin to come out of isolation.[64]

Early in the pandemic, the public health message of "flattening the curve" proved effective, leading to the shutdown of public places to ensure that hospitals did not become overwhelmed. During the government shutdown, hospitals planned measures to increase their surge capacity, improve management strategies, and acquire more PPE. However, the indefinite closure of certain industries placed thousands of people in a precarious financial position. Increased economic pressure prompted local and state governments to begin reopening the economy, which expectedly led to an increase in cases. Though several states in the United States placed restrictions on the amount of people allowed in various establishments, these guidelines quickly became impossible to enforce.[65] Furthermore, a substantial number of people are also refusing to wear masks when in public, further exacerbating the current spread of disease.[66] In these situations, HCWs have a responsibility to the general population to advocate for public health measures. Most people are not on the front lines and cannot see the direct impacts of the current pandemic. HCWs should share their knowledge and experiences with others to encourage proper social distancing, hand hygiene, and mask wearing among the general public.

Given these conditions, it is no surprise that a second wave of infections is threatening to overwhelm hospital systems. In some projections, the second wave appears to be positioned to lead to more infections than the first. In Houston, Texas, home of the largest medical center in the world, the cases dramatically increased after reopening businesses, threatening ICU capacity.[67] Interestingly, it appears that this second wave of hospitalizations is made up of a much younger patient population than the initial wave.[68] This suggests that public health messaging likely needs to be improved to reach younger individuals who may feel that the virus is not likely to cause them serious harm. Hospitals and clinicians have made substantive progress in rising to the challenge posed by COVID-19; however, ultimate control of this virus is likely going to require the coordinated efforts of government, public health officials, and health-care systems.

Conclusion

The COVID-19 pandemic has created various challenges for HCWs. As health-care institutions and governments struggled to control the first wave of infections, HCWs were placed in situations where their own health and safety came into conflict with their desire to serve their patients. Many were forced to make personal decisions about whether to continue to work during this pandemic, and those that stayed were faced with significant ethical dilemmas never faced before in their careers. Furthermore, the continuously changing guidelines and the limited PPE availability have placed an extra strain on HCWs in terms of their ability to protect themselves and their families at home. The mental and emotional burdens of being on the front lines of the COVID-19 response will likely need to be continually managed for the duration of the pandemic. While initially overwhelmed, health-care systems have rapidly adapted, from increasing access to PPE to improving planning for patient surges. Overall, as a result of this pandemic, HCWs have seen a shift from their primary roles from being clinicians to also being educators, researchers, and public health advocates.

References

1. Li Q, Guan X, Wu P, et al. Early transmission dynamics in Wuhan, China, of novel coronavirus-infected pneumonia. *N Engl J Med*. 2020;382:1199–1207.
2. ICN - International Council of Nurses. *More Than 600 Nurses Die From COVID-19 Worldwide*; 2020. [online] Available at: https://www.icn.ch/news/more-600-nurses-die-covid-19-worldwide. Accessed 3 July 2020.
3. Chan PS, Berg RA, Nadkarni VM. Code blue during the COVID-19 pandemic. *Circ Cardiovasc Qual Outcomes*. 2020;13(5), e006779.
4. Bruzda N. *COVID-19 And The Ethical Questions It Poses. [online]*. University of Nevada Las Vegas; 2020. Available at: https://www.unlv.edu/news/release/covid-19-and-ethical-questions-it-poses. Accessed 3 July 2020.
5. Vergano M, Bertolini G, Giannini A, et al. Clinical ethics recommendations for the allocation of intensive care treatments. In: *Exceptional, Resource-Limited Circumstances*; 2020. Available at: http://www.siaarti.it/SiteAssets/News/COVID19%20-%20documenti%20SIAARTI/SIAARTI%20-%20Covid-19%20-%20Clinical%20Ethics%20Recomendations.pdf. Accessed 30 June 2020.
6. Rosenbaum L. Facing Covid-19 in Italy - ethics, logistics, and therapeutics on the Epidemic's front line. *N Engl J Med*. 2020;382(20):1873–1875.
7. DeFilippis EM, Ranard LS, Berg DD. Cardiopulmonary resuscitation during the COVID-19 pandemic: a view from trainees on the front line. *Circulation*. 2020;141(23):1833–1835.
8. McGrath BA, Brenner MJ, Warrillow SJ, et al. Tracheostomy in the COVID-19 era: global and multidisciplinary guidance [published online ahead of print, 2020 May 15]. *Lancet Respir Med*. 2020. https://doi.org/10.1016/S2213-2600(20)30230-7.
9. American Medical Association. *AMA Code Of Medical Ethics' Opinion On Physician Duty To Treat. [online]*; 2020. Available at: https://journalofethics.ama-assn.org/article/ama-code-medical-ethics-opinion-physician-duty-treat/2010-06#:~:text=Because

%20of%20their%20commitment%20to,own%20safety%2C%20health%20or%20life. Accessed 3 July 2020.

10. Murphy B. *COVID-19: States Call On Early Medical School Grads To Bolster Workforce. [online]*. American Medical Association; 2020. Available at: https://www.ama-assn.org/delivering-care/public-health/covid-19-states-call-early-medical-school-grads-bolster-workforce. Accessed 3 July 2020.

11. Society of Critical Care Medicine (SCCM). *COVID-19: Calls For Volunteers. [online]*; 2020. Available at: https://www.sccm.org/Disaster/COVID19/COVID19-Calls-for-Volunteers. Accessed 3 July 2020.

12. Gallegos A. *Concerns For Clinicians Over 65 Grow In The Face Of COVID-19. [online] Medscape*; 2020. Available at: https://www.medscape.com/viewarticle/928488. Accessed 3 July 2020.

13. Buerhaus PI, Auerbach DI, Staiger DO. Older Clinicians and the Surge in Novel Coronavirus Disease 2019 (COVID-19) [published online ahead of print, 2020 Mar 30]. *JAMA*. 2020. https://doi.org/10.1001/jama.2020.4978.

14. Tian J, Yuan X, Xiao J, et al. Clinical characteristics and risk factors associated with COVID-19 disease severity in patients with cancer in Wuhan, China: a multicentre, retrospective, cohort study. *Lancet Oncol*. 2020;21(7):893–903.

15. Richardson S, Hirsch JS, Narasimhan M, et al. Presenting characteristics, comorbidities, and outcomes among 5700 patients hospitalized with COVID-19 in the new York City area [published online ahead of print, 2020 Apr 22] [published correction appears in doi:10.1001/jama.2020.7681]. *JAMA*. 2020;323(20):2052–2059.

16. Neale T. *An Age/Old Dilemma? Pulling Senior Cardiologists From The Front During COVID-19. [online] TCT MD*; 2020. Available at: https://www.tctmd.com/news/ageold-dilemma-pulling-senior-cardiologists-front-during-covid-19. Accessed 30 June 2020.

17. Menon V, Padhy SK. Ethical dilemmas faced by health care workers during COVID-19 pandemic: issues, implications and suggestions. *Asian J Psychiatr*. 2020;51:102116.

18. Hanto DW. What should I do? *Ann Surg*. 2020. https://doi.org/10.1097/sla.0000000000004007. Publish Ahead of Print.

19. Rosenbaum L. Once upon a time…the Hero sheltered in place [Online ahead of print]. N Engl J Med doi:https://doi.org/10.1056/NEJMp2015556.

20. Wu Z, McGoogan J. Characteristics of and important lessons from the coronavirus disease 2019 (COVID-19) outbreak in China. *JAMA*. 2020;323(13):1239.

21. Medscape. *In Memoriam: Healthcare Workers Who Have Died Of COVID-19. [online]*; 2020. Available at: https://www.medscape.com/viewarticle/927976. Accessed 22 June 2020.

22. Centers for Disease Control and Prevention. *Coronavirus Disease 2019 (COVID-19) In The U.S. [online]*; 2020. Available at: https://www.cdc.gov/coronavirus/2019-ncov/cases-updates/cases-in-us.html. Accessed 3 July 2020.

23. Gondi S, Beckman A, Deveau N, et al. Personal protective equipment needs in the USA during the COVID-19 pandemic. *Lancet*. 2020;395(10237):e90–e91.

24. Jessop Z, Dobbs T, Ali S, et al. Personal protective equipment (PPE) for surgeons during COVID-19 pandemic: a systematic review of availability, usage, and rationing. *Br J Surg*. 2020.

25. Rosenbaum L. Harnessing our humanity—how Washington's health care workers have risen to the pandemic challenge. *N Engl J Med*. 2020;382(22):2069–2071.

26. Santarpia J, Rivera D, Herrera V, et al. *Aerosol and Surface Transmission Potential of SARS-CoV-2*; 2020 [MedRXIV].

27. Ong S, Tan Y, Chia P, et al. Air, surface environmental, and personal protective equipment contamination by severe acute respiratory syndrome coronavirus 2 (SARS-CoV-2) from a symptomatic patient. *JAMA*. 2020;323(16):1610.

28. Guo Z, Wang Z, Zhang S, et al. Aerosol and surface distribution of severe acute respiratory syndrome coronavirus 2 in hospital wards, Wuhan, China, 2020. *Emerg Infect Dis*. 2020;26(7):1583–1591. https://doi.org/10.3201/eid2607.200885.

29. Fang Y, Zhang H, Xie J, et al. Sensitivity of chest CT for COVID-19: comparison to RT-PCR. *Radiology*. 2020. Published online February 19.

30. West CP, Montori VM, Sampathkumar P. COVID-19 testing: the threat of false-negative results. *Mayo Clin Proc*. 2020;95(6):1127–1129.

31. Ip DKM, Lau EHY, Tam YH, So HC, Cowling BJ, Kwok HKH. Increases in absenteeism among health care workers in Hong Kong during influenza epidemics, 2004-2009. *BMC Infect Dis*. 2015;15. https://doi.org/10.1186/s12879-015-1316-y. 586-586.

32. Krystal J, McNeil R. Responding to the hidden pandemic for healthcare workers: stress. *Nat Med*. 2020;26(5):639.

33. Monica FPE, et al. Preparation and response to COVID-19 outbreak in Singapore: A case report. *Infection Disease Health*. 2020. https://doi.org/10.1016/j.idh.2020.04.002.

34. Centers for Disease Control and Prevention. *Coronavirus Disease Return-To-Work Criteria. [online]*; 2020. Available at: https://www.cdc.gov/coronavirus/2019-ncov/hcp/return-to-work.html?CDC_AA_refVal=https%3A%2F%2Fwww.cdc.gov%2Fcoronavirus%2F2019-ncov%2Fhealthcare-facilities%2Fhcp-return-work.html. Accessed 30 June 2020.

35. Tate C. *Hilton, Marriott Donate Free Hotel Rooms For Medical Workers Responding To Cornavirus Crisis [online]*. USA Today; 2020. Available at: https://www.usatoday.com/story/travel/2020/04/12/coronavirus-hilton-marriott-give-free-hotel-rooms-medical-workers/2978567001/. Accessed 30 June 2020.

36. Brown. *Brown Provides Short-Term Residence Hall Housing To Front-Line Personnel Fighting COVID-19. [online]*; 2020. Available at: https://www.brown.edu/news/2020-04-21/residence. Accessed 30 June 2020.

37. Deam J. *Rice University Will Open Its Residence Halls To Health Care Workers Fighting The Coronavirus. [online]*. Houston Chronicle; 2020. Available at: https://www.houstonchronicle.com/news/houston-texas/houston/article/RICE-RESIDENTIAL-HALLS-15180793.php. Accessed 30 June 2020.

38. Britto B. *University Of St. Thomas Offers Empty Residence Hall Rooms To Hospitals. [online]*. Houston Chronicle; 2020. Available at: https://www.houstonchronicle.com/news/education/article/University-of-St-Thomas-offers-empty-residence-15183096.php. Accessed 30 June 2020.

39. Tufts Now. *Tufts To Make Residence Halls Available To Local Hospitals And Host Cities. [online]*; 2020. Available at: https://now.tufts.edu/articles/tufts-make-residence-halls-available-local-hospitals-and-host-cities. Accessed 30 June 2020.

40. Vimercati L, Tafuri S, Chironna M, et al. The COVID-19 hotel for healthcare workers: an Italian best practice. Published Online Ahead of Print, *J Hosp Infect*. 2020.

41. NIH. *Litcovid. [online]*; 2020. Available at: https://www.ncbi.nlm.nih.gov/research/coronavirus/. Accessed 3 July 2020.

42. Corsello D, Gotur D, Carroll C, Masud F, Simpson S. Impact of small-N studies during a pandemic. *Chest*. 2020. https://doi.org/10.1016/j.chest.2020.05.581.

43. Miller DG, Pierson L, Doernberg S. The role of medical students during the COVID-19 pandemic [published online ahead of print, 2020 Apr 7]. *Ann Intern Med*. 2020;M20-1281. https://doi.org/10.7326/M20-1281.

44. Hester TB, Cartwright JD, DiGiovine DG, et al. Training and deployment of medical students as respiratory therapist extenders during COVID-19. *ATS Scholar*. 2020;1(2): 145–151.

45. Goshua A. *Medical Students Called To The Covid-19 Fight Need Protection. [online]*. STAT News; 2020. Available at: https://www.statnews.com/2020/04/17/medical-students-called-covid-19-fight-need-support-protection/. Accessed 5 July 2020.

46. Lapolla P, Mingoli A. COVID-19 changes medical education in Italy: will other countries follow? *Postgrad Med J*. 2020;96(1137):375–376. https://doi.org/10.1136/postgradmedj-2020-137876.

47. Pugh R. *COVID-19: Medical Students' Fast Track Plans Finalised. [online]*. Medscape; 2020. Available at: https://www.medscape.com/viewarticle/927628. Accessed 5 July 2020.

48. Murphy B. *Residents Share Fears, Views On Training Disruptions During COVID-19. [online]*. American Medical Association; 2020. Available at: https://www.ama-assn.org/residents-students/resident-student-health/residents-share-fears-views-training-disruptions-during. Accessed 5 July 2020.

49. Ronan L. *[Online] Residency Training in the Era of COVID-19: A Program Director Weighs in*; 2020. Available at https://in-housestaff.org/residency-training-covid-19-program-director-1675. Accessed 5 July 2020.

50. Lagoe A. *Going Full-On Macgyver' – U Of M Doctor Creates Makeshift Ventilators To Battle COVID-19. [online] Kare 11*; 2020. Available at: https://www.kare11.com/article/news/health/coronavirus/going-full-on-macgyver-u-of-m-doctor-creates-makeshift-ventilators-to-battle-covid-19/89-ecf8ced9-fd76-478b-ad6e-ae3aeab50b4a. Accessed 5 July 2020.

51. University of Utah. *Innovation In Response To COVID-19. [online]*; 2020. Available at: https://uofuhealth.utah.edu/center-for-medical-innovation/blogs/2020/03/covid-update.php#revised-aerosol. Accessed 5 July 2020.

52. Ross C. *Debate Flares Over Using AI To Detect Covid-19 In Lung Scans. [online] STAT*; 2020. Available at: https://www.statnews.com/2020/03/30/debate-over-artificial-intelligence-to-detect-covid-19-in-lung-scans/. Accessed 5 July 2020.

53. Holmes R. Is COVID-19 social media's levelling up moment? *Forbes*. 2020. Available at https://www.forbes.com/sites/ryanholmes/2020/04/24/is-covid-19-social-medias-levelling-up-moment/#7f6ff6ac6c60. Accessed 5 July 2020.

54. Ahrens E. *How COVID-19 has changed social media engagement. SproutSocial. Available at*. https://sproutsocial.com/insights/covid19-social-media-changes/. Accessed 4 July 2020.

55. Li HO, Bailey A, Huynh D, et al. YouTube as a source of information on COVID-19: a pandemic of misinformation? *BMJ Glob Health*. 2020;5, e002604.

56. Anoruo NA. How social media undermined the COVID-19 response. *ABC News*. 2020. Available at https://abcnews.go.com/Health/social-media-undermined-covid-19-response/story?id=70511613. Accessed 5 July 2020.

57. Ahmad AR, Murad HR. The impact of social media on panic during the COVID-19 pandemic in Iraqi Kurdistan: online questionnaire study. *J Med Internet Res*. 2020;22(5), e19556.

58. Gautret P, Lagier JC, Parola P, et al. Hydroxychloroquine and azithromycin as a treatment of COVID-19: results of an open-label non-randomized clinical trial. *Int J Antimicrob Agents*. 2020. Available at https://www.sciencedirect.com/science/article/pii/S0924857920300996?via%3Dihub. Accessed 5 July 2020.

59. Griffiths J. *Wuhan is the latest crisis to face China's Xi, and it's exposing major flaws in his model of control.* CNN; 2020. Jan 24. [online] Available at: https://www.cnn.com/2020/01/23/asia/wuhan-china-coronavirus-sars-response-intl-hnk/index.html. Accessed 2 July 2020.

60. Bremmer I. The Best Global Responses to COVID-19 Pandemic. [online] Available at. Time https://time.com/5851633/best-global-responses-covid-19/ [Accessed 2 July 2020].

61. Pisano GP, Sadun R, Zanini M. Lessons from Italy's response to the coronavirus. *Harv Bus Rev.* 2020. [online] Available at: https://hbr.org/2020/03/lessons-from-italys-response-to-coronavirus. Accessed 2 July 2020.

62. Francescani, C. Timeline: The First 100 Days of New York Gov. Andrew Cuomo's COVID-19 Response. Available at. ABC News https://abcnews.go.com/US/News/timeline-100-days-york-gov-andrew-cuomos-covid/story?id=71292880. [Accessed 3 July 2020].

63. Rossman J. Herd immunity in Europe - are we close? *The Conversation.* 2020. Available at https://theconversation.com/herd-immunity-in-europe-are-we-close-139253. Accessed 3 July 2020.

64. Fiore K. *Are Stockholm's Hospitals About to Break?* Medpage Today; 2020. Available at https://www.medpagetoday.com/infectiousdisease/covid19/86256. Accessed 3 July 2020.

65. Barned-Smith S. *311 Calls Report Social Distance Violators Everywhere From Swing Sets To Adult Novelty Shops. [online].* HoustonChronicle.com; 2020. Available at: https://www.houstonchronicle.com/news/houston-texas/houston/article/coronavirus-calls-social-distancing-porn-shops-311-15176972.php. Accessed 30 June 2020.

66. Weissert W, Lemire J. *Face Masks Make A Political Statement In Era Of Coronavirus. [online].* AP NEWS; 2020. Available at: https://apnews.com/7dce310db6e85b31d735e81d0af6769c. Accessed 4 July 2020.

67. Nuila R. *The Coronavirus Surge That Texas Could Have Seen Coming. [online].* The New Yorker; 2020. Available at: https://www.newyorker.com/science/medical-dispatch/the-coronavirus-surge-that-texas-could-have-seen-coming?utm_source. Accessed 30 June 2020.

68. Cha A. *Younger Adults Are Large Percentage Of Coronavirus Hospitalizations In United States, According To New CDC Data. [online].* Washington Post; 2020. Available at: https://www.washingtonpost.com/health/2020/03/19/younger-adults-are-large-percentage-coronavirus-hospitalizations-united-states-according-new-cdc-data/. Accessed 30 June 2020.

Allocating scarce medical resources: Inequity in the face of crisis (in pursuit of PPE)

Marilia Díaz[a,b] and Jacqueline Y. Steuer[c,d]

[a]*Hospital Auxilio Mutuo, San Juan, Puerto Rico,* [b]*Universidad Sagrado Corazón, San Juan, Puerto Rico,* [c]*Manager Critical Care Services APN team,* [d]*NorthShore University HealthSystem, Evanston, IL, United States*

Early in March of 2020, everything changed in the intensive care units (ICUs) throughout the nation. All of the sudden, surgical and N95 masks were the most valuable items in a hospital. Everyone wanted to have a spare few of them to make sure they will have some while working. Since then, having enough personal protective equipment (PPE) is like hitting the jackpot. It gives a sense of security and control.

Either you were prepared for the first coronavirus disease 2019 (COVID-19) patient or not. Even if prepared, no one would have never imagined what was going to happen. Uncertainty was in the air. Most probably, everyone has read about past pandemics while in the college but nothing could prepare anyone enough for what was coming. There was a job to do and it was going to get done, but deep down everyone was scared.

It is March 11, 2020 in a 26-bed ICU at a tertiary hospital in a 5-hospital system. Everyone is being shuttled out of the halls. Corridors shut off. Visitors told to stay in the rooms. Patients' doors and curtains closed. Staff buzzing around. A room set up for emergent intubation and line insertion. Drips ready: pressors, intravenous fluids, sedation. Vent on, settings in place. Nursing, respiratory therapy, intensivist, and anesthesia in full PPE). The nervous energy is palpable. The fear is tangible. People are afraid—staff, patients, and visitors. Only staff know what is really going on, but families and patients know is something big. In rolls the first COVID-19 positive ICU patient. Decompensated on the medical floor in less than 12 h. The patient needs to be intubated. Like a well-orchestrated routine, the patient is positioned on the ICU bed, quickly sedated, intubated, lined, and drips started. And so, it begins.

Same day, a 23-bed ICU, but the story is completely different. The first COVID-19 patient is already in the ICU, but no one knows he has the virus. Now, what? How does staff take care of him? What changes in patient care needs to be done? The patient has been in the ICU for days; now, every nurse and physician who has been taking care of the patient is scared. No plans were made before that day.

COVID-19 Pandemic. https://doi.org/10.1016/B978-0-323-82860-4.00003-3

Decisions needed to be made and fast. Should we take the intravenous pumps out of the room? Does the treatment need to be changed? What happens to the other patients in the ICU? Did staff get exposed? Are they sick? Will they get sick? There are a lot of questions and little time to make the best decisions possible.

Many in North America have been preparing for this COVID-19 pandemic since early January. Witness to the situations in other countries put plans in motion early. A novel virus. So highly contagious because the body does not recognize it as ill causing. Those facilities that had not been preparing; well, they were not so well equipped. Frankly, even those who planned were not so well equipped at times. Some areas were hit much harder with cases than others. Italy, Seattle Washington and the New York City had devastating number of cases and deaths. Illinois fared fairly well, as did some other midwestern states in the US. Some areas of the world did not heed the warnings of resurgence, as a number of positive cases were dropping and in other areas significantly rising. So begins a record-breaking number of cases in new areas. Some in politics didn't believe this was going to be a problem and shared their belief. This encouraged people to flock to certain places which resulted in markedly increased cases of COVID. Schools and restaurants closed because those areas wanted to reduce the spread of COVID. Businesses closed. Home schooling? Who ever thought of that? All businesses struggled, except alcohol sales. They skyrocketed. That 5-hospital system mentioned in the beginning of the chapter, well they began preparing the second week in January… and they had issues too. Everyone did. Equipment was scarce, and PPE was nearly impossible to come by in the early days.

On March 13, everything changed on the island as in many other places. In a blink of an eye, lives as health-care workers changed. A new virus is spreading and fast. Outside the hospitals, it was a complete chaos. Long lines at the supermarkets and warehouses just to buy the essentials to be prepared for the lockdown. People bought surgical masks, N95 masks, gloves, face shields, and any kind of disinfectant cleansers. Staff feared hospitals wouldn't be able to buy more supplies because of the worldwide high demand. Every single day, going to work at the ICU thinking that will there be enough supplies to get through the pandemic? Now, plans are also needed to have PPE secured. There were patients in isolation, not because of COVID-19, and they required care as well. Organization was the key. Nursing activities had to be more productive, to take care of patients safely, and to properly use the PPE. Even the most experienced ICU nurse can forget something needed for a task, yet no one could afford to waste the PPE. Working together as a team approach was needed more than ever. A motto was used: "together we can beat the virus."

What was happening in hospitals?

Well, that depends where? New York City had so many cases so fast, they ran out of equipment, let alone PPE. Staff ended up contracting the condition, some of whom died. Critical care communities all over the world, for the first time, were talking to each other and sharing ideas. Social media was the fastest way to share experiences, what worked and what did not. What a frightening time, and yet the proudest time to be in health care. Government support was crucial. That was not always there. Some leaders understood the concern and supported the needs of health-care organizations. Some did not. Some called this a fake pandemic. Some claimed to have done a great job getting a handle on this pandemic… some of those might have been the same people who originally called this pandemic fake. Not all political leaders led by example. Some did. Not all recognized the PPE issues, some did. The health-care providers certainly did. Did the public? Some did and some did not.

Hospitals began filling up fast. So did ICUs. Requests for hand gel, a new mask and more gowns were met with, this is what we have. There is direction to reuse the mask. Organizations are out of gel, so hand wash. In the COVID units, use the gown patient to patient. This was happening everywhere. Those not in health care were in a panic. Buying up toilet paper, bleach wipes, and hand gel like there was no tomorrow. There was such a high demand for health-care grade PPE, and organizations were going through products so fast, shortages occurred. Worse yet, employees of some organizations were found to be stealing PPE to sell on social media platforms for their own financial benefit or stealing for their own personal use. This time brought out the worst and best in people.

After days of hearing about the lack of hand gel, bleach wipes, and masks, the community got together. There were requests on social media from friends and families of health-care workers, and health-care workers themselves first asking, then begging for home donations of "any" products to give to hospitals and first-line responders. It happened in the Midwest, east, and west coasts, internationally. People began making masks in which a filter could be placed into it. Vacuum high efficiency particulate air filters ran out of stock. Truckloads of supplies were delivered to hospitals. Some hospitals allowed the use, some did not. Those frontline workers felt however anything was better than nothing. The support from the public was unsurmountable. Everyone felt like "we are in this together."

Why was PPE so hard to obtain? This was known to be coming. Hospitals were preparing and ordering supplies like crazy. Suddenly, there were no supplies to be had. Manufacturers were out of masks, gowns, and gloves. No hospital-grade germicidal wipes or sprays were available. Hand gel could not be found. How does this happen? Politicians knew this was coming. Health-care experts knew this was coming. Hospitals knew this was coming. How come manufacturing did not? Or could they simply not keep up with demand? Nearly 4 months after that first patient rolled in, bleach wipes could not be purchased for household use. Hand gel still hard to come by. So much so that liquor manufacturers began making hand gel and giving, yes giving, it away to health-care workers and first-line responders. How does this happen in North America, South America, Europe? Areas of excellent health care are really struggling. Other areas of the world are not. Why the discrepancy? Or is everyone struggling to obtain supplies and some are just not vocal about it? The Governor of the New York State was on the TV every day. He speaks of shortages and how supplies are being shifted from one area to the next. How grave the need is! Some politicians still debunk what is happening. How can this be? A record number of people are dying. Famous people have contracted this disease and said, this is no joke. This is no flu. Why can't people get what they need?

Surgical masks had always been single use. Once they are moist, they need to be changed. So single use it is. Now, people are told to wear a surgical mask for a week or longer. Keep it in a pocket. Reuse it until visibly soiled. There are suggestions to keep the mask in a brown paper bag. It dries out faster, and there is less chance of contaminants growing in paper than stored in plastic bags. Paper breaths and hopefully this works to protect people in health care. Is something better than nothing?

N95 masks used for particular respiratory infections including COVID-19 are typically a single use. Again, the message is the same as the surgical mask. Wear indefinitely. Keep it in a paper bag, add a name on it, so as not to use someone else's. If a COVID unit, it stays in the equipment room. If not a COVID unit, take it with even in a multihospital system. Again, is something better than nothing?

Why did this happen? Why the sudden change in practice? For over 30 years, this equipment is single-patient or daily use. Now use until it can't be used anymore.

Gowns made of plastic or bunny suits are to protect the wearer. In the COVID units, the staff is wearing a gown room to room. This was never done before. Yet, there does not seem to be any bad outcomes with this practice. Was health care wasteful before? Is health care more prudent now? Is this impact of a shortage teaching valuable lessons? Everyone is doing this across the globe. Why? Because something is better than nothing. Or are there issues simply do not know about? Suddenly, gowns are back to single-patient use. Is it because supply is up? Or is there an issue? Time will tell, as there is more retrospective information to come.

Replacement gowns are shabby, like plastic wrap. Stronger, better made gowns are needed. These cheap gowns tear almost by a breath. The fear of self-contamination is ever present. This is all that is available? Workers refuse to wear, suggest the administrators do. Material managers are told to find quality gowns. They show up. Administrators and material managers are grateful to get their hands on any products, some of which however are subpar. They simply don't realize it. It is unfortunate. It takes the frontline worker to say, this won't work. Support is there. They agree. But are the gowns there? Eventually. Hopefully, no self-contamination!

Gloves. Wear two pair. After a patient is examined, remove the outer pair. Clean the pair underneath with hand gel, re-apply a new pair. Go to the next patient. Really? This is being done around the globe. Some don't even wear two pairs, just one. Consequences? None so far thankfully. Again… something better than nothing.

Clean hands are the mainstay of any infection control issue, including this pandemic. Historically, the plan is clean hands with gel between touching anything. In the room, gel hands. Touch the patient, gel hands. Touch the computer, gel hands. Gel on the way out. Now, a new practice. Gel on the way in and after removing the outer gloves on the way out. Thankfully, no obvious consequences. Wasteful before? Not certain. For now, better than nothing?

Powered air purifying respirators are also known as PAPRS. There won't be enough for everyone, so they are reserved for those who are in the COVID units for extended periods of time. What? How is this possible? The PAPRS are used so often, they begin to break. Some units have a great supply. Some ICUs and emergency departments (EDs) have barely enough. How does this happen? How can anesthesia have PAPRS for their entire teams, including transport and ICU, and ED can only get for those with extended periods?

Initially, everyone needs a N95 mask. Oh wait, there is another change. There are not enough N95 masks for everyone. New plan. Everyone in the ICU and ED needs a N95 mask for patient care. Outside of these areas, N95s are needed only if the patient has a lot of coughing. Isn't that the main symptom of this infection? If no significant coughing, a surgical mask on the patient as well as the staff is sufficient. Since when?

What happened to flatten the curve? Well, it all depends on where you live. Some places managed to flatten the curve and others didn't. The ones who flattened the curve were able to manage better the shortage of PPE. Relying on others, like the government, to flatten the curve is merely impossible. Education and common sense are the way to go. Less patients mean more PPE available for a longer period of time, and no one knows when COVID-19 will be out of our lives. Less patients also mean less exposure for health-care workers. There is no need to manufacture more PPE if less people get infected. We don't need more PPE factories; we need less exposure which translates into less patients.

The World Health Organization states masks won't help. The Centers for Disease Control says it does. Why the controversy? People are confused. Staff are confused. The impetus for the mask is to slow down the droplets likely by about 70%. So, less droplets, less virus transmission. The end result is that to wear a mask in public to reduce droplets and in hospitals at all times. Were health-care organizations wasteful before the reuse of masks? Did health care create its own shortage because they were not thoughtful about PPE use? Did providers utilize PPE above and beyond because of fear, and this make a shortage even worse. Is single use really the answers, until there is a shortage, and then the rules change? In the same scenario, what would be desired for PPE? All of it. The desire would be all of it. Is that understandable? Hell yes. Did health care learn something? Unsure. There are no consequences easily found of reuse. Will practice change? Time will tell.

Providers were confused. Messages changed often. They needed PPE to protect themselves and their families at home. The recommendations on the PPE use changed often. Why did this happen? Were organizations better informed? Was in response to shortages? Both? Likely both.

Providers were frustrated. They wanted employers to protect them. Employers were frustrated. The ability to get supplies was a 24 h a day job. Employers really were doing their damnedest to get PPE. Material Managers were working tirelessly with distributors. No one wanted anyone unprotected. Things became available on the black market. There was price gouging. Were certain supplies legit? There were donated supplies. Its ok for use in home, but not in the hospitals? Suddenly, it's OK to use donated supplies? It's the only option. Because something is better than nothing.

In addition to the nervous fatigue about PPE availability, providers experienced other issues. The PPE was hot. It didn't matter what: bunny suits, plastic gowns, gloves, N95s, and/or PAPRs. Breathing was OK but not normal. Some experienced anxiety. Sounds were muffled. Sounds were difficult to hear. Phone conversations, well they were impossible. Trying to talk on the phone to a consult or family in PPE did not work. Staff required breaks. There were skin breakdown, rashes, and blemishes. Staff were tired. They felt an increase in fatigue and exhaustion. PPE certainly contributed. Staff were afraid, hungry, and frustrated. Yet, back in they went, in full PPE.

Providers were concerned about self-contamination. No one wanted to bring this home to their families. Were they even protected with reused PPE? Apparently so, as so few medical personnel was exposed and suffered dire consequences. There were some that were, but most were not. Can this change practice in the future? Can garbage load on the world be reduced with less plastic gloves, gowns? Maybe? Maybe not? Did this pandemic teach us anything about practice and waste? Certainly yes. Will it change practice. Well, time will tell.

What will be the long-term effect of the use of PPE on providers? Will there be some type of PTSD? Hopefully not. But that won't know for a while. Will staff become more reactionary to latex and other plastic products? Hopefully not. But that won't be known for a while either.

Patients also experienced a significant difference in their patient/provider relationship. They no longer could appreciate the genuine, reassuring smile from their health-care providers. They saw eyes, covered by face shields. They felt separated, and they were. Speaking to patients who recovered from COVID, they felt like a leper. They were bustled into exam rooms; they were seen virtually from home; they were separated from everyone whether inpatient or outpatient. They felt isolated from the health-care community. Yet, they were grateful for the care and concern. Those inpatients, they were alone, some of them critically ill. There was no human touch, no skin to skin. It was glove to skin. Even Florence Nightingale spoke of the need for skin-to-skin contact. None of that for staff or patients during this time. Providers stated that they just wanted to hold the hand of a dying patient. Not through a glove. They wanted the last thing that patient felt as they left this earth, was the human touch. Not possible. And as health-care workers, there is grave sorrow for that. Who suffered more? Likely both.

For years, health-care workers in the ICU have been incorporating the presence of the family in the ICU and seeing them as part of the team, but now, they are no longer welcomed in the hospital. Now, patients are alone in their rooms. Are we not allowing any relatives because of the shortage of PPE or because everyone is scared of COVID-19? Anyhow the social aspect of this will likely contribute to significant trauma to patients and staff worldwide. The staff who just wanted to hold that dying persons hand... not gloved... but didn't because of fear. The patient who in hospital or at home was isolated. Not really experiencing the contact of the provider–patient relationship as it is known because it is separated by physical barriers. Most staff develop relationships with their patients that includes touch. Not here, not now.

Everyone is grateful for the work people put in worldwide to obtain PPE to protect frontline workers. How can this be better, God forbid, there is a next time? Political leaders "need" to rely on their experts, listen to their experts, and make factual statements. A plan must be put into place immediately. A well-needed plan in place not needed is better than one not in place and needed. This is not a blame game, but a work together game. Politicians need to work together with health-care experts for a plan that is thoughtful and beneficial for all. The public needs to heed warnings and take them seriously. During pandemic is a time to put the health of all citizens as top priority. This is not a political issue, but a social issue. Everyone is responsible and accountable.

The proudest moment truly was the sharing of ideas, thoughts, and practices in health care worldwide. What a proud moment for all health-care workers! Experts and bedside clinicians dialoging with those in China, Europe, North and South America, Africa, and Australia. What worked? What didn't? How were these situations handled? What a consortium! There was no race to be the first. It was working together to handle this. What a proud moment!

In the pursuit of PPE, PPE is much more available worldwide. Many health-care organizations have gone back to old practices, some have not. Bleach wipes and disinfectant sprays however are still not available for personal use. That will come. When everyone has a moment to think, looking at practices for PPE use should be examined. Maybe that worldwide consortium again? Can the garbage load for the world be reduced if everyone did a certain practice? Likely. Most important to remember, the PPE use in hospitals and in public is not political, its social and an important thing to remember. Stay safe all and be well.

COVID-19 and risk exposure of the front line: Heroes or martyrs?

Marilia Díaz

Hospital Auxilio Mutuo, San Juan, Puerto Rico, Universidad Sagrado Corazón, San Juan, Puerto Rico

Are we heroes or martyrs? Well, it depends on many things. At the beginning of the pandemic, everyone saw us as heroes and I even came to feel like one. But in movies, superheroes are not afraid of anything, and we are afraid of infecting ourselves and infecting our relatives.

Social media was saturated with videos showing everyone's appreciation to health professionals. Television advertisements also thanking us for our hard work and dedication. Multiple movements were formed to applaud health professionals at night in appreciation for being on the front line of the battle against coronavirus disease 2019 (COVID-19). On social media, people shared photos and drawings of doctors, nurses, respiratory therapists, and cleaning staff with phrases acknowledging their heroic activity or dressed as superheroes. Singers dedicated songs to fans who work in hospitals. Artists appreciated in their pages the work done. Stores offered discounts and even free food. We did not have to queue in the stores, and they thanked us for the service we were giving. Don't get me wrong, all of those actions even brought me to tears. It was a little bit of happiness in a world full of chaos. But the days passed and then the weeks and little by little, we began to be forgotten.

But in other parts of the world, it was a very different experience from the start of the pandemic. Social media showed videos and news of nurses who were being discriminated against. People did not want to share the elevator or the stairs with them in residential buildings or public places. Random people left them notes on their doors indicating that they could not continue living there. Others threw chlorine at some nurses while they were trying to use public transportation. Even vehicle drivers would not allow them to get into their cars. In addition to all of this, remember to add the long continuous hours of work. Sometimes they had to work up to 24 h in the hospital.

And what about the use of personal protective equipment (PPE)? Well, it all depends on where you work. Working in a COVID unit or in the emergency room means wearing PPE during the entire work shift. Social media has presented us with the faces of health-care workers full of marks from the use of PPE. Those marks not

COVID-19 Pandemic. https://doi.org/10.1016/B978-0-323-82860-4.00016-1

only remain on the faces but will also remain in their memory. Do you think wearing the mask while shopping is annoying? That's about 1 h or less of use. Now remember that work shifts are 8 h or more. Those are 8 continuous hours wearing N95 masks that lacerate cheekbones, septum, and chin. The worst thing is that they work several days a week, so frequent use causes lacerations, and the next day you have to use the same fitted mask that you have to put on over the laceration. The fear of contagion is so great that we work without removing the mask, so we do not drink water, and now, we have another additional problem, dehydrated personnel. Before many came to their work shifts with their water bottles which they consumed before the end of the shift but now it is different. What is better to live a little dehydrated or get infected?

And not to mention the clothing. It does not matter if you only wear a plastic robe or a coverall, you will feel very hot when using it. After working for 30 min caring for a patient, you are all sweaty, and so we have to stay like that the rest of the shift, because there is no time to lose. You may ask yourself, doesn't they have air conditioning at the hospital? Yes, but the amount of PPE and the material it is made of is like being in a plastic bag for hours. This adds to the already dehydrated staff working at the hospitals. It is surely a hazard to all of health-care workers.

Long working hours and the number of patients to attend to are no longer the same as before, one can say it has doubled and, in some places, even tripled. The first few weeks of the pandemic, people did not want to go to the hospital unless it was more than necessary; they thought they could get COVID-19 while there. This caused that in the hospitals where only a few patients but as the cases of COVID-19 increased, the emergency rooms began to fill patients with all the suspected cases of COVID-19. Little by little the hospitals began to fill with patients, and the staff did not give time to take care of all of them. The intensive care units began to fill with the COVID-19-infected patients who were in worse condition. The task of proning a patient has never been easy, but now, we have to do it with all the PPE on. On top of it, all of those who didn't take good care of themselves for months now are arriving at the hospitals too sick.

These big quantities of work hours wearing a mask and proper PPE at first looked just like a warning of what was to come, for some meant rethinking, am I fit for the job? Did I study the right thing? I can contaminate someone? To many nurses this came as a shock, some weren't willing to go through this, as so there where many nurses who where up to the job even though they were scared. I mean they are humans; I believe humans are the most vulnerable creatures of this world because they are exposed to all impurities that surround them, and COVID-19 came not only as a life lesson demonstrating not only how fragile life is but how our minds function and how emotions play a big role in our lives. Those nurses who decided they were not fit for this job are not considered weak, but instead what demonstrates is the mind playing defense mechanism.

Professional interrelations were affected, and differences in opinion came in and shook the minds of those who wanted to be in the front line. Some thought that they were not being rightfully protected by their institutions, and there came the problems, there came the real tears. Everyone had a different opinion, they were not all on the same page, the institutions and all the leaders were so stressed, they had this "hurricane category 5" on top of them that it was difficult to think straight right. COVID-19 was a novel thing, and they had no previous clue of how to protect humanity, it doesn't matter where do you live, the impact would be imminent, and it's already here. Now, they were so centered on planning how to manage that they forgot about the stress bomb forming underneath them, the staff was full of insecurities and fear, and it had to be addressed as top priority. What should the institutions address first the need for PPE or the fear of the staff? Both things are equally important, but it was easier to look for PPE than to take care of the staff emotions. That's why many of the staff called in sick for days and even for a whole month, they wanted to make sure that the correct PPE was available before going back to work. Who can blame them? Maybe you think that we are heroes because we are the first line of defense, but what if I tell you that we are not only afraid but also tired. The long hours of work take a toll on us. We weren't mentally prepared for this, and the worst part is, we are mentally exhausted, yet, we are doing our job and trying to survive during this pandemic. But as days goes by, we are dealing with it better, the support from coworkers, relatives, and friends helps to get us through, and social media is a wonderful way to stay together.

This pandemic not only affects emotionally nurses, it affects doctors too. On March, the first health-care professional, a nurse, got infected. The doctor explained to her that she needed to be intubated. That moment affected everyone in the intensive care unit. The natural thought was that could be me. At that moment, the only thing I wanted to do was to tell my family how much I love them. I wanted to get out of the shift, I didn't want to take care of my patient because she is my coworker, and I was devastated by looking at her getting sicker. I knew I needed to be there for her, she needed me as her nurse and I knew that mentally I could do the job. Right there it hit me, I had to forget my emotions and do the job. As nurses we go through so much stress, it is unbearable at times. We are working with lives, and saving people is our number one priority, so many people depend on us. Seeing her intubated and not getting any better stranded nurses and doctors in the hospital. Every single time any of us took a look at her though that could be any of us. Heroes don't get scared, heroes don't cry, and heroes are strong. Now, I no longer want to be a hero.

Seeing patients getting better gives me hopes in humanity and life. Not everything is lost, it gives me the strength I need to go back to work every day and be a better health-care professional and a good coworker. Coping has many stages, and COVID-19 have us going through all of them. COVID-19 not only came as a virus but also to teach us how vulnerable we can be and how important it is to constantly educate ourselves and evolve. Changing will get us through this pandemic. Every day is a new lesson to learn. We will rise wiser and stronger like the superheroes.

Talk about being a health-care worker and a teacher at the same time, it was truly stressful. After a long day at the hospital, now, it is the time to be a parent. How can someone who is mentally exhausted can help a child with the schoolwork? I think after this, the true heroes are the teachers. Teaching multiplication to a child can be painful as being on your feet for 8 h and harder than getting a peripheral intravenous into a dehydrated patient. Tell me that is not overwhelming but trying to be a health-care professional, a parent, and a teacher? This proved to be too much, but at the end, we have been able to do it.

Protocol? Is there a protocol? Who do we follow? I mean Centers for Disease Control and Prevention places a new protocol every day and a new thing every time you open a computer? World Health Organization is all so popping and cooking COVID-19 information and standards. Every time an infectologist comes through the door they have a new plan to try, whether it is vitamin C by loads, remdesivir, convalescent plasma, proning a patient, I mean I understand all, but it feels like a race to see who does better, who wins the race. As all of this runs through my mind, the word "protocol" is right behind. Every time my supervisor calls a huddle and she starts with, I know this is all hard on us, the next thing I hear is "protocol" in my mind because I know that something and somebody new came up with a new thing that we are going to try and that not only gives me goosebumps but gets me in tears and I want to run and cry, but at the same time, I just take a deep breath and say to myself "let's do this, you got this."

COVID-19 vs health-care system that is our reality. Health vs economy? Can you only imagine what could happen if this wave of patients keeps on going up? The economy is important, but life is too. Are health-care workers heroes or martyrs? You have the answer in your hands. Taking care of yourself and your family from exposing to COVID-19 is the way to go. I will be your hero when you get sick and I take care of you. If you expose yourself to COVID-19 and get infected, I will be a martyr taking care of you, but at the same time, fearing I could get contaminated from you.

Are we really heroes? Are we treated as heroes? Heroes always overcome evil but we have already lost a lot. At the beginning of the year, I saw news from China and Europe where health professionals were dying from COVID-19. It saddened me to know that so many were dying, but at the same time, I was wondering, how is this possible? Those are the kind of things that must see to believe. Sadly, the time came when I had to see a colleague die. On that day, many of us cried including doctors, nurses, and respiratory therapists. The sadness was felt in the environment which later became into fear. No one goes to work in search of death, we work for the health of many, but now, it is ours that is in danger. That day we realized how vulnerable we are to this virus. The days passed, and the news about the deaths of doctors and nurses around the world continued. People gave up their lives to combat COVID-19. We don't want to lose more health professionals in this battle.

The obligatory question is, do we want to be heroes or do we want to be martyrs? I think we don't want to be either. Each professional wants to be appreciated for their work, but in the same way, they want to be able to do it safely. We want to have the right PPE that protects us well and not use what "is better than nothing." The best way to protect health professionals is by following the recommendations of the experts. It is necessary for the population to avoid becoming infected, and this is achieved with physical distancing, the use of a mask, and frequent hand washing. There are three simple actions that we must take to stop this virus, and that no other health professional ends up being a martyr to the pandemic.

Do I believe in humanity after quarantine? As a human I believe that as an adult and as a nurse I do think that we need to educate our present and future about prevention, which is the most important base of all. If you educate, you can help to stop the spread of any infection that comes in our way. Life as I see it is based on prioritizing, and it should be based on having a constant education. Education is the base, and we should be responsible for our own education and for educating our families and the whole community. And how do we do this? Here is my answer, one person at a time, that's the way. Building trust is never easy, and right now, humanity has lost trust in a lot of things, and they only believe what is tangible or their own life experiences, unfortunately, that is the reality in many homes around the world. Now, our responsibility is to rebuild that trust. As health-care providers, we should not only be the ones who rebuild that trust, but first, we should be able to work on ourselves, that is caring for the provider. Our peers can help us to do so. We share so much time together and have so many things alike that we can understand each other. There could be another pandemic or a natural disaster, but we all have the ability to be a hero again, we need to build our strength.

COVID-19 and social media

Patxi Pérez Fernández[a] and Miguel Moreno Aríztegui[b]

[a]*President, The Association of Journalists of Navarra, Pamplona, Spain,* [b]*Advisor, The President of the Government of Navarra, Pamplona, Spain*

Introduction

Beware of false prophets, which come to you in sheep's clothing, but inwardly they are ravening wolves

Matthew 7:15

The original severe acute respiratory syndrome coronavirus 2 (SARS-CoV-2) also known as coronavirus disease 2019 (COVID-19) spread from China to other neighboring countries to then relentless reach Europe, Italy, and Spain first, and later the United States and the rest of the World. Initially thought to be a different form of flu, drawing increasing media attention in February 2020 was soon to be declared a pandemic by the World Health Organization (WHO) in March 11, 2020 changing the world situation and creating a surreal scenario that continues up to date. Media interest towards the health situation was in crescendo. Data coming from health authorities, official organisms, scientists and experts were showing signs of concerns on the rapid rise of infectiousness in the population. Journalism took the position as witness and herald of the communication and discovery of risks associated to the virus and the historical milestones created by a health emergency have never experienced before. And then, it came the confinement, the social alarm in some countries where governments struggled to enforce policies and emergency laws while trying to maintain a decent socio-economic environment. The financial turmoil affected also the press and the media, as some newspapers and communication companies ordered their staff to telework, closing newsrooms and offices, along what was being experienced in other aspects of life such as schools and business in general. The world stopped in disbelief. The COVID-19 pandemic assaulted us by surprise, unprepared, and uncovered miscoordination of agencies and entire governments.

But a worse enemy was yet to be discovered: disbelief, human arrogance, and vested interest. These factors accompanied and altered many decisions, information, and policies and determined actions that would lead to major changes in our way of life.

85

In this historical scenario, and more than ever, journalism has given the role and responsibility to be the herald of the information for the public. COVID-19 pandemic has served as a motive for media evolution. Freelancers and war journalists have turned into video calls, home reporting, and "out-of-field" communication. The dynamics of journalists have changed, and in some instances, the reach to the reader or listener has evolved in a way that maintaining rigor and accuracy has become a challenge by itself.

The essential role of the journalists in the society rests in their ability to present facts and contrasted information without bias or influences. But social networking and multimedia platforms present the risk of easy mass transmission of unfiltered information. The appearance of these modern communication methods has brought the option of delivering non-contrasted information to the public. How to know what information is or is not a hoax? How to contrast news or information? Can we eradicate the so-called "fake news"?

The concept of "fake news" is deceiving by itself. The meaning of "news" implies to be truthful. That is to say, the word "news" by its definition carries veracity of what is told, and therefore we should not deteriorate the concept "News-News" with the adjectives "true or false". Therefore once referring to "fake news" the term false information or hoax must be kept handy.

During the pandemic, we have witnessed an outbreak of hoaxes and out of context information in health, drug industry, politics, finances, and government policies, together with many indirectly associated but related issues such as police actions, protests, nutritional support, and environmental requests.

Media plays a crucial role in creating a globally informed society, and journalism carries the responsibility of playing that role. It is exactly that professional attitude is an important quality that separates true journalist from writers of the news or facts, as it was reflected in the words of the Minister of Defense of the Spanish Government, Margarita Robles: "Journalism is more necessary than ever and citizens value its public service role. They are the oxygen of democracy, their role as informants, and public opinion makers makes them essential. For this reason, at this time is when it is more necessary for the media to exercise journalism responsibly, providing information of general and proven interest."[1]

The digital transformation of the media. A compromised quality?

COVID-19 pandemic has marked a paradox for media companies around the world: while the coronavirus outbreak has drawn attention and there has been a significant increase in news consumption, the economic impact of the crisis has forced the companies to accelerate their digitization and to reduce their workforce.[2]

The pandemic has not done but, as in so many other sectors, accelerate changes that would have occurred in the same way, but more slowly. "The bottom line is that we see an accelerating movement towards digital media and media on mobile devices and various types of platforms," says Rasmus Kleis Nielsen, the director of the Reuters Institute. "This is accompanied by a continued decline in confidence in the news and a growing concern about misinformation, particularly on social media and by some politicians."[2]

The business prospects for media corporations are not good: when most of them had still not managed to recover from the 2008 crisis, there is another dramatic drop in advertising revenue. Around the world, leading newspapers have opted for subscriptions for their digital platforms. For most companies, this has become an essential source of income to sustain their independence and maintain their plurality.[3]

The difficult task now lies ahead of convincing readers that independent press is not synonymous with free press, and that subscription modalities are a need, not a donation. The aforementioned drop in revenue from conventional advertising and the cannibalization of revenue that social media platforms do with media-generated content have created a critical situation, forcing publishers to insist on the cost of creating news under high journalistic standards. In the opinion of Adrienne Lafrance, deputy director of *The Atlantic*, "it will be crucial to diversify the sources of income although a subscription model ensures you a base of readers that value what you do best." Lafrance believes that this "vicious circle" reinforces "the need to serve the public while encouraging quality journalism."[2]

The so-called philosophy of "everything for free" installed on the Internet has proven unfeasible for media with high-quality standards. The increasing quantity of information does not reflect pluralism by itself, but rather a dramatic decrease in quality: junk information and "clickbait," as denounced by José Miguel Mulet Biochemistry and Molecular Biology professor at the University of Valencia and renowned scientific divulgator.[4]

Paywalls

Media corporations are betting into direct subscriptions as way of financing. This method separates the practice of the most common digital platforms that offer free content and subsidize their operations with advertising.[5]

There are several models for financing media companies, all sharing the common denominator of seeking independence from advertisers and agencies and establishing a link with their readers. The traditional advertising model has been falling for years, and everything indicates that this year it will do so even more: according to a report by IAB Spain and PwC, most sectors have cut their advertising investment in digital media as a result of the coronavirus crisis.[6]

Paywalls can be divided into five types:

Closed—simply pay to enter the newspaper's website or media website and consult any type of news item, regardless of its type or relevance.

1. Partially closed—it consists of closing a part of its content, the most important and high quality, in exchange for a subscription or registration. Current or less exclusive contents are open to any reader. This model is the most commonly used by different media sources.

2. Limit of readings—it allows a limited number of readings or limits the number of words by article or content. When the limit is reached, the subscription is requested. This is becoming the most popular pay limiting system.
3. Dynamic—the combination of several types of paywalls. They can choose to open some articles and close others while, the website obtains information of the reader, choosing the right moment to offer the subscription and or exposing them to "targeted advertising."
4. Support or advantages—uses the need for independence as the motive and request the reader to support the media to avoid advertising. Essentially, it is a pay for eliminating advertisements. It can also include additional advantages such as subscriptions to other media, access to online sources, etc.

Social media and hoaxes

A great part of the digital transformation of the media is the appearance of social networks, nominated as winners of the dissemination of hoaxes. This is one of the conclusions reached by a group of researchers from the University of Navarra and the Barcelona Supercomputing Center, when analyzing the health hoaxes disseminated during the first month of state of alarm in Spain.[7]

Hoaxes about the coronavirus are being disseminated mainly on closed messaging platforms or social networks, especially on WhatsApp. It has also been observed that counterfeit content is detected, as the pandemic, in addition to generating a large number of hoaxes about health and science, it has also facilitated the dissemination of numerous false political and financial claims.

Hoaxes on science and health issues are often generated in foreign grounds, while those of political nature although using the pandemic as a noisy background are typically domestic in origin. Identity theft is a common mechanism in hoaxes: they try to deceive citizens by making them believe that their content originates in credible institutions or authorities. Some hoaxes might be close to become fraudulent and concerns exist about their potential use as a weapon to create financial instability.

According to the mentioned study, hoax is defined as "all content that is intentionally false and appears to be true, conceived in order to deceive the public, and publicly disseminated by any platform or social communication medium." It also establishes a typology in which four types of hoaxes are identified: joke, exaggeration, decontextualization, and deception. From these four types, the researchers propose a "diagram of the severity of hoaxes," which indicates them as more serious the higher level of falsehood and willfulness in their dissemination.

The dissemination of hoaxes and information of a xenophobic and offensive nature on social networks began to force multinationals to position themselves. In June 2020, The Coca-Cola group placed all its advertising on social media on hold for at least 30 days, a move that was followed by several companies in the wake of racial protests in the United States and the rest of the world. According to CNBC,

James Quincey, CEO of Coca-Cola Corporation stated: "… We will use this period to reassess our advertising policies and determine what revisions are needed. We also expect greater accountability and transparency from our partners in social networks." "There is no place—he added—for racism in the world, and there is no place for racism on social networks."[8] The company explained that the measure was to in support of the boycott to Facebook promoted by various civil rights organizations. The suspension of paid advertising on social networks was also announced by the Unilever group, manufacturer of brands such as Dove, Ben & Jerry's and Hellmann's, as well as the Levi Strauss & Co.

Enrique Dans, an expert in communication and technology, points out examples of the dangers of viral transmission of messages in social media, as occurred in India in 2018 where several attacks took place in different areas of the country after messages forwarded by WhatsApp that warned against alleged networks of people who tried to kidnap children to sell their organs. After that, as reflected by the Indian newspaper *Business Standard*, Facebook limited the forwarding of messages in WhatsApp, decision that has been accompanied by more than 70% reduction in the dissemination of potentially dangerous messages.[9]

The value of true information

We previously stated the concern that the public has regarding the veracity of the information. In a similar fashion, the journalist must be always in the search for contrasting the confirming sources and details. That cannot be done without a major investigational effort. Searching and researching is the only way to provide accurate and contrasted information. A rigorous analytical process must prevail as the executional mode for true journalism. From the media corporation standpoint, resources and time must be placed at the disposal of the journalist, while securing external sources that will allow for the contrast of information. As all this comes to a cost, and considering the difficulties associated with the current pandemic and the financial shortages that most media have experienced, it is not uncommon that some news might hit the public without the completeness process that they pertain. Those "fake news" hit the audience provoking repercussions at all levels of the society.

Therefore journalism must be not only the guarantor of the news but also the prosecutor of the "fake news." In May 2020, the United Nations launched an initiative named "verified" to fight against "fake news" advocating at the same time for a serious source verification and contrasting any news regarding the pandemic. Mr. Antonio Guterres, the Secretary-General of the United Nations, affirmed that "we cannot give up our virtual spaces to those who traffic in lies, fear, and hatred. Disinformation spreads online, in messaging apps, and from person to person. Its creators use intelligent methods of production and distribution. To counter it, scientists and institutions like the United Nations need to reach people with accurate information they can trust."[10]

The initiative is centered around three areas of information:

- Health and science—to save lives;
- Solidarity—to promote local and global cooperation; and
- Solutions—to advocate for support to affected populations.

To guarantee this project, the United Nations has made a call for global volunteers to register as informants enabling them to provide and share information with friends and family. This process will form a myriad of information teams, described as digital emergency teams. These volunteers will receive a daily verified information content package that can be easily shared helping the fight against fake news while filling information gaps.

The project will partner with influencers, civil authorities, businesses, the media, and social media to distribute its content and to help to extinguish harmful claims about COVID-19.

Even prior to this pandemic, the European Union (EU) had worked on the transcendence of bad information or intentional hoaxes and tried to establish instruments to counteract its proliferation.

During the pandemic, more than ever before it has become evident that the cost of being misinformed is too high. For a long time, it has been taken for granted that noninformed people were misinformed due to lack of access to the truth. However, it is becoming more evident that it is due to an excess of circulating misinformation. Truthfulness and information have become commodities as scarce as "drinking water amid a flood."

True information comes not only by the description of the facts but also on the contextualization. As stated by Marta García in *El Confidencial*, our impulse to believe certain things is stronger that our capacity to change our opinion. This is even more noticeable in our rapid changing environment. Then it is growingly important to understand that the fight against misinformation cannot be fought with simple facts and headlines.[11]

Tools against false information

Everything said above, the verification of the news to date passes through the rigor of the professional. However, ensuring the truthfulness of the information is as important as guaranteeing that false news do not get published, for which anticipation is required. For that reason, in an attempt to provide resources beyond the human professional alone, some platforms have emerged. One of them, Eventum contracts people to verify news and data and applies advanced algorithms to reduce and eliminate fake news. In tests carried out on its alpha network, the Eventum platform managed to identify stories with "fake news" in less than 3 min. As explained by Martín Milken, one of the partners of Eventum: "Our network uses a combination of three elements: incentivized collective collaboration (crowdsourcing), an advanced algorithm, and blockchain technology. The combination of the three allow us to detect false news quickly and cheaply."[12]

Policies and regulations

Even before the pandemic, a major concern existed among members of the EU regarding "fake news." Addressing this issue, the European External Action Service was created by the year 2015. It was formed by a group of over thirty experts, including senior journalists, representatives from news organizations, academicians, and experts in facts verification. The group was in charge of assessing and regulating actions of the media and press. One of the first actions of this Task Force was to survey the public in general. During the months of November 2017 to February 2018, a public consultation was held for citizens included a phone survey that reached over 26,000 citizens. Up to 83% of the survey responders considered fake news a danger to democracy and 37% of them confirmed finding fake news on a daily basis. In the same survey, 45% of the responders believed that journalists were responsible for the transmission of the fake news, while 39% believed that such responsibility fell into the governments and 36% on the news corporations.[13]

The EU, with advice of the experts, defined four principles to guide the action against fake news: transparency (origin and sponsorship of the source), diversity of the sources, credibility, and inclusiveness (allowing all interested parties to participate). These principles marked the origin of the Code of Good Practice. Besides the adherence to the four principles previously described, the code calls for prosecuting fake accounts in social media and prioritizing true content news in search engines and other channels. In the search for success, it is essential to have the compromise of the big search engines and social media platforms, a compromised obtained shortly after.[13]

The work needs to continue in the eradication of the misinformation. One of the solutions was the creation of SOMA (Social Observatory for the Misinformation and Social Media Analysis). The objective of this institution is to support experts in their work against misinformation by providing them with a useful infrastructure and connecting them to a broad community of peers to collaborate on specific tasks. Other projects include the Rapid Alert System, with a purpose to monitor and detect misinformation affecting the institutions or its members. The goal of this project is, through the collaboration among member nations, to avoid false campaigns and the spread of hoaxes while sharing good practices with other international organizations.

Of interest is to analyze the types and effects of hoaxes. A group of researchers from the University of Navarra and the Barcelona Supercomputing Center have analyzed the typology of hoaxes disseminated in Spain, from March to April 2020. The results, published in the journal "*El profesional de la Information*," indicated the finding of 292 hoaxes in the three Spanish platforms accredited by the International Fact-Checking Network: Maldita.es; Newtral, and EFE Verifica. Most of the false statements were spread mainly through text messaging (53.8%), the most basic and easy to manipulate format. Although less frequent, numerous hoaxes based on multimedia formats were also detected—photo (25.6%), video (14.6%), and audio (5.7%)—whose presence was somewhat more frequent on open networks such as Twitter. This team of researchers concluded that the use of audiovisual in combination with other formats or content was preferred by the hoaxers. In fact, it was common to find real photographs and videos that are decontextualized by means of a text that falsely attributed them to particular events or place.[14]

Four categories of hoaxes were identified: jokes, exaggerations, wrong context, and deception. Deception, simply defined as false information, was unquestionably the most frequent modality of hoax (64.4%). Slightly, more than half (97 of the 188 hoaxes) found in the sample resorted to identity theft; that is, in order to give them greater credibility, they attributed their content to reputable sources, often trademarks. Beyond seeking the simple confusion of the citizenship, some of the deceptions had the purpose of economic fraud.

Wrong context (17.1% of hoaxes) was frequently linked to photographic or video formats: real images, often months or even years prior, that are falsely attributed to a noncorresponding context. For example, a photo shared on social media showing dozens of coffins line up in Italy attributed to deaths from the coronavirus pandemic, but in reality, the photo was related to an incident occurred in the year 2013, involving a major drowning of sub-Saharan immigrants who drowned while trying to reach the shores of Lampedusa.

Exaggeration (17.1%) was detected in several areas, especially in the political debate. Exaggeration is, for example, a hoax launched by Pablo Echenique Robba, the deputy spokeperson for "Unidas Podemos," a leftist political party in the Spanish Parliament, accusing the right-handed party, Vox, of breaching the confinement orders and sending all its representatives (52) to the congress, while in reality only 16 of them had attended the sessions and were within the regulations and ordinances.

With just 1.4% of the total, the least frequent hoax modality in the sample studied was jokes. This type corresponds to "that type of hoax that consists in the dissemination of false information, with a burlesque, parodic, satirical, or cartoonish purpose."

Scientific sources to verify information

The coronavirus pandemic has shown the importance and value of scientific advisory for the media. Health and science advisors are increasingly needed to stand by political leaders. While realizing that we were not prepared for a health crisis like the one we are experiencing and after witnessing the improvisation, sometimes lack of organization and misled political decisions by governments and institutions, the importance of the presence of a scientific board in our institutions, including media corporations, becomes more evident than ever.

Many scientific institutions including universities, hospitals, laboratories, and pharmaceutical companies have redoubled their efforts to make available technologies and human resources to health authorities. But the scientific community is not exempt of the same communication problems and ethical dilemmas as the rest of the world. Sometimes moved by impulse, or the wish for results or even political motives, information could be biased or even falsified. In the late May and early June 2020, shortly after the president Trump wrongfully attributed a value to hydroxychloroquine that was out of range, many voices were risen in the scientific community against this message and attempts to deviate or halt its use in the treatment of COVID-19. Again, some "unfiltered information" against the president Trump's claims was made available and even published in well-respected medical journals. Right after, a major scandal was uncovered, shaking the foundations of the scientific system from the base to the top. *The Lancet* and the *New England Journal of Medicine* had both published articles deeming the inefficiency and risks associated to hydroxychloroquine in the treatment of COVID-19, to later discover the biased interest of some of the authors as well as the unsupported and non-contrasted results presented. Both journals have to retract their publications, an event seldom seen in the recent history of both publications.[15]

However, the deed caused by these articles was not minor. Shortly after the publication and without time for response or contrasting analysis, the WHO suspended all trials that included the drug on any arm and soon the treatment disappeared from its use. It was later that different articles and the voice of scientists from Australia and some from the United States questioned the results published in these two journals causing the investigation and discovering that non-contrasted data and flaw results were included, modifying the results and the drawing of false conclusions. By that time, damage was already done, and hydroxychloroquine was no longer used or favored by the scientific community and the bad atmosphere around it made it tremendously difficult to conduct further unbiassed or blinded studies.

A similar but in the opposite side of the coin was the ivermectine, an antiparasitic drug that according to one investigation reduced the mortality rate of COVID-19 patients by up to 83%. Although it was a "preprint"—a preliminary result without expert review—published in April on the SSRN platform. Its publication had a major impact in Latin America causing a widespread use of the medication in Peru, Bolivia, or Dominican Republic.[16]

As we get closer to the development of a vaccine, these types of misleading events call for a very cautious scientific evaluation and advice prior to the publication of any news.

There are additional nonhealth-related consequences of the opinions generated by a health opinion body. Information about new treatment developments, failures, or successes as well as advisory related to the movement or activities of the population can impact the economy and even the political trend of a country. Considering that there is a proliferation of front pages and continuous media interviews, reports, and opinions of scientists, these have turned into major influencers, and their "genuine exposure" and lack of experience in communication make them sometimes an easy target for producers and scriptwriters.

The creators of false news often use the anonymous source methodology in which the issuer is not disclosed, and logically, the information is not supported by a legal source or individual. Hence, it is not unusual that when investigating the hoax, noticeable characteristics of those are the source being unknown to the public, enhanced academic positions for the source or a loaded curriculum for the speaker, or a given appearance as a solvent entity. In the mentioned study, only 4.1% of the hoaxes came from fictitious sources. An example is the video in YouTube titled "The Coronavirus can be stopped in 24 hours," attributed to an alleged graduate in molecular biology, Isidro Fuentes García, a person who does not really exist.[17]

Maybe because information collected in social networks is more difficult to control than that appearing on traditional media, statistics and numbers are notably more frequent, now, especially with the pandemic. Multiple notes appear regarding the origin and lethality of the virus, its permanence in the environment, treatments, or vaccines. Frequently, we see false recommendations or treatments for virus (gargles, diets and wine, homeopathy, or the "miraculous mineral supplement"). To a lesser extent, falsehoods related to health management in hospitals and facilities are also found, as well as hoaxes spread by health assumptions or falsely attributed to public health institutions, such as the WHO.

The digital and technological platforms and the power of the networks

European and US platforms, as well as for most countries, depend in great part on foreign countries for their actuation, cybersecurity, or storage. The technological dependence opens risks in relation to property, privacy, and data protection as well as in implementation of innovation projects. Policies aimed to protect and to make these networks independent are being developed by both the EU and the United States. As stated by Margrethe Vestager "there is a conviction that in the EU it is necessary to ensure its digital technological sovereignty in key areas, so as not to depend on other economic areas in something that is so essential and strategic. Even before COVID-19, this was one of the priorities of the European Commission. The epidemic has only accentuated it, and this will lead the EU to act on at least three fronts." Those three fronts can be summarized as data infrastructures, regulatory changes that guarantee sovereignty, and rules to regulate competition (fair balance). Some experts have seen the digital platforms as the great beneficiaries of the coronavirus pandemic. Indeed, during the states of exception and confinement around the world, e-commerce using any of the digital support platforms has increased volume by several folds. This has been the perfect environment for large technology companies to imbed themselves along the households of many citizens. According to Reuters, European Press Agency, these are large technology companies, mostly private, with global operations and little regulation. In many cases, their business is based on accessing their user's personal data. The lack of regulations on accessing data gives them an incalculable comparative advantage compared to other types of businesses, more traditional and not exclusively digital, which, however, are subject to regulation.

The politicians' influence

The Trump's effect on Internet has been notorious. First, he was criticized as not following the traditional channels to communicate with the public and rather using Twitter to transmit critical information. Later, this practice has been adopted by many mandataries airing the question on why this is happening. Why are governments bypassing traditional media to inform public in general? Maybe the answer is the accessibility or maybe is just the need to bypass intermediaries. Some authorities have mentioned the advantage of the speed and free of opinion of the direct methods of information. However, the use of social media is not exempt of problems. Many messages can be rapidly labeled and targeted with counter campaigns. Messages and rumors mix with news and hoaxes and rapidly spread throughout the world. Venezuela's president Nicolás Maduro has accused the United States to instigate rebellion and coups, Iranian chief of the revolution Ali Khamenei has called for the destruction of Israel among others.

President Trump voiced out his intentions to reform the Section 230 called Communications Decency Law, approved in 1996. It is also a fact that for years, politicians, journalists, and editors of all kinds of media have been demanding precisely this regulation to be reformed. An excerpt of the law: "No provider or user of an interactive computing service may be treated as an editor or issuer of any information from another information content provider." Based on US jurisprudence, this means that social networks are not responsible for the content that is published on them, no matter how false, injurious, or criminal it may be. Even the democrat candidate for the 2020 presidential election, Joe Biden agree with the intention of the reform. In the words of president Trump, "when the big and powerful social network companies censor the opinions with which they do not they agree wield dangerous power... Online platforms are engaging in selective censorship that is harming our national discourse."

It is to be seen however if this regulation of the digital platform comes to a benefit to the traditional media which might need to consider their methods in order not to be excluded from their ultimate goal of communicating news. Press and democracy have walked together for the past two centuries. It is likely that we will see a different world after COVID-19. As the frailness of the health system has been exposed by the pandemic, the weaknesses and failures of the media network have been seriously manifested, and there is uncertainty on the survival of some of them.

How to control the media and information

The control of the media has been sought by politicians, economists, businessmen, and even public personalities. Woodrow Wilson, US President during the World War I spread a strategy using the press to gain support among the citizenship has involved the United States into the big war. In a similar way, the role of the press and radio networks during World War II was essential in Churchill's leadership. Later on, press and media, by then including TV, played a major role throughout the Cold War era.

The big media corporations are not just TV or press but they cross different scenarios, and some are involved in the financial and investment world. For example, Microsoft is a leader in informatics and digital media. The diversification of these groups makes them very difficult target with regard to controlling them, and although this might be a good point, with regard to press independence, it is a dangerous motive of concern.[18] While media groups try to guarantee their information with the credibility and rigor of their professional journalists, there is fear of the possibility of using information and direct to consumer platforms as weapons. How can we control this threat? Natalia Sara explains that "this is the VUCA context (volatility, uncertainty, complexity, and ambiguity) … in the face of misinformation and falsehood, a company must act by communicating what the truth or the facts are and transmit them to all its stakeholders and, depending on the case, denounce the wrongful us if it."[19]

Negative news is shared much faster than positive ones. Anything that generates noise forces you to be more proactive, report it, and validate it. One of the things that have made this crisis unprecedented is that, for the first time in history, an "infodemic" has been declared. There have been days in which more than 600 hoaxes about COVID-19 have been published. The misinformation has been total. It has been predicted that by 2022, social networks and digital platforms will contain more false than real information. This leads us to the fact that companies must make greater communication efforts. At the same time, we should promote consumer responsibility.

Media can be controlled but information must not be. The utopian possibility of controlling information goes through the difficulty of enclosing ideas, opinions, and news in a box and that has been and is being tried by totalitarian governments, dictatorial systems, and even the capitalist system. This must not happen and we, the press, have the ultimate tool to prevent it: information.

References

1. *Libertad Digital*; 2020.
2. *Digital News Report*. Reuters Institute; 2020.
3. https://es.reuters.com/article/entertainmentNews/idESKBN23N1AJ.
4. Mulet JM. *Que es la vida Saludable?* Spain: Ediciones Destino; 2019.
5. https://www.elconfidencial.com/el-valor-de-la-informacion/2020-06-17/periodismo-muro-pago-democracia_2639428/.
6. Forte F. *Coronavirus impact on digital advertising investment by sector Spain 2020*. Statista; 2020. April.
7. https://www.unav.edu/web/facultad-de-comunicacion/detalle-noticia2/2020/05/21/un-estudio-de-los-bulos-sobre-la-covid19-confirma-que-las-social-networks-are-your-main-environment-of-diffusion-above-the-journalistic-media/-/asset_publisher/ngL9/content/.
8. *Coca-Cola pauses advertising on all social media platforms globally*; 2020. https://www.cnbc.com/2020/06/26/coca-cola-pauses-advertising-on-all-social-media-platforms-globally.html?__source=sharebar|email&par=sharebar.

9. *How WhatsApp Destroyed A Village.* https://www.buzzfeednews.com/article/pranavdixit/whatsapp-destroyed-village-lynchings-rainpada-india.

10. Guterres A. *Secretary General of the United Nations in a statement.* Dated 21 May; 2020.

11. Aller MG. *Article in the digital El Confidencial.* 18 May; 2020.

12. https://www.prnewswire.co.uk/news-releases/fighting-fake-news-with-blockchain-new-eventum-platform-detects-bogus-content-in-minutes-684135691.html.

13. https://www.europarl.europa.eu/RegData/etudes/STUD/2019/608864/IPOL_STU(2019)608864_EN.pdf.

14. Salaverria R, Busion N, et al. Desinformación en tiempos de pandemia: tipología de los bulos sobre la COVID-19. *El profesional de la Información.* 2020;29(3):e290315. https://doi.org/10.3145/epi.2020.may.15.

15. Joseph A. Lancet, New England Journal retract Covid-19 studies, including one that raised safety concerns about malaria drugs. *STATS.* 2020. PARS International Corp.

16. Caly L, Druce J, et al. The FDA-approved drug ivermectin inhibits the replication of SARS-CoV-2 in vitro. *Antiviral Res.* 2020;178. https://doi.org/10.1016/j.antiviral.2020.104787, 104787.

17. Amautell A. *El bulo de que el dióxido de cloro cura el coronavirus.* Sociedad; 2020. https://www.65ymas.com/sociedad/bulo-dioxido-cloro-cura-coronavirus_14008_102.html.

18. Hendriks P. Expansion strategies of newspaper firms: diversification and innovation. In: *Newspapers: A Lost Cause?* Dordrecht: Springer; 1999. https://doi.org/10.1007/978-94-011-4587-9_5.

19. Sara N. *jscomunicaciondecrisis.com.* March; 2020.

COVID-19 and the role of medical professional societies

Drew Farmer[a], Jose Pascual[a], and Lewis J. Kaplan[a,b]

[a]*Perelman School of Medicine, University of Pennsylvania, Division of Trauma, Surgical Critical Care and Emergency Surgery, Philadelphia, PA, United States,* [b]*Society of Critical Care Medicine, Mount Prospect, IL, United States*

Introduction

Membership in a medical professional organization, or society, is both voluntary and common. Many clinicians belong to more than one such society, especially if they practice critical care medicine. They belong to one or more organizations related to their parent discipline, as well as related to the subspecialty of critical care medicine. Each of the memberships comes at a financial cost. Moreover, membership in a specific society often leads to service for the organization as part of a committee, taskforce, or workgroup. For some, this service paves a path to medical professional organization leadership as well. The latter path is true of two of this chapter's authors. Recognizing that leadership is much less common than organizational service, it is appropriate to explore what benefits members derive from membership in a medical professional society as part of their regular professional life. Given the pandemic that currently grips the globe, it is equally important to explore the role of medical professional organizations within that context as well.

Medical professional organization types

In general, medical professional organizations exist as six broad types: (1) those related to parent discipline or subspecialty certification (e.g., American Board of Medical Specialties[1]); (2) those joining or aligning individuals who trained in a specific parent discipline (e.g., American Society of Anesthesiologists[2]); (3) those joining or aligning individuals who trained in, or practice within, a specific subspecialty or care for a specific patient type [e.g., Society of Critical Care Medicine (SCCM)[3]]; (4) cross-specialty organizations focused on a specific condition or set of events (e.g., American Red Cross[4]); (5) nongovernmental organizations that deploy members to locations for disaster relief or to address crisis conditions (e.g., Médecins Sans Frontières[5]); and (6) governmental organizations that utilize volunteer experts in

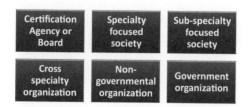

FIG. 1

Types of medical professional organizations.

addition to full- or part-time medical professionals (e.g., Centers for Disease Control and Prevention[6] and World Health Organization[7]). Each of these organization types serves a function for members and in turn are served by them (Fig. 1).

Member benefits

Since no one is mandated to join a medical professional organization—even if one must utilize the services provided by one such as those comprising the American Board of Medical Specialties—membership must confer benefits perceived to be of value by members. This is particularly true since there is a financial cost to membership that recurs each year. Many members are bereft of a funding stream from their employer to secure membership and therefore pay out of pocket. Multiprofessional organizations embrace members who have widely divergent salary streams. While some have a single membership cost, others, such as SCCM, have developed a tiered membership strategy that supports joining at different price points, albeit with different accompanying benefits. Regardless of membership type or price, members of medical professional organizations enjoy benefits that are common to most such organizations (Fig. 2).

First, members enjoy linkage with other members with similar interests. This commonly occurs at yearly meetings but also occurs within committees for which members may volunteer. Second, committee membership allows members to work with others toward a common goal, augment their experience, expand their curriculum vitae, and learn leadership skills. Third, committee work may also guide one into a leadership role within the committee, further developing a skill set that translates into the member's workspace as well. Fourth, some multiprofessional organizations have groups comprised of individuals with a similar parent training discipline (i.e., internal medicine as opposed to nursing). Those groups, often termed sections, offer the same parallel opportunities for member's work, education, skill acquisition, and leadership as does volunteering for the larger organization.

Fifth, members typically receive a medical professional journal (known as the official organ of the society) as well as newsletters and related educational communications. Each of these provide venues for new knowledge transfer, controversy identification and debate, as well as notification of upcoming events. Sixth, in

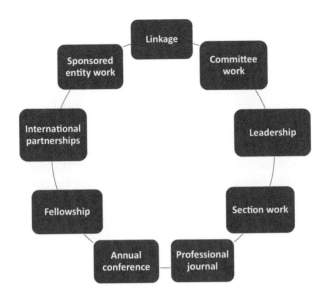

FIG. 2

Member benefits.

addition to networking opportunities as noted earlier, most organizations host an annual conference, meeting, or congress, that is educationally focused, often reveals cutting edge-research, may teach new skills, or offer review courses to support member professional development in a socially satisfying context. Seventh, many organizations also host a pathway to being recognized as having reached a career milestone. While some utilize a parallel structure termed a "college" within which to house that pathway, the clinician who reaches that milestone earns the designation of "fellow." In general, there are specific criteria that need to be met, an application is required, and a committee who reviews applicants and submits recommendations to a governing body with whom the ultimate authority rests to confer fellowship. Achieving such status also supports reappointment and more often promotion with the academic community. In this way, highly regarded honors may be achieved during the course of one's membership. Other awards are often conferred for unique achievement or exceptional service as well.

Eighth, some organizations also partner with others within the same country, providing yet another way for members to participate in, and learn about related organizations besides within the annual meeting. An apt example is the Critical Care Societies Collaborative comprised of the American Association of Critical Care Nurses, the American College of Chest Physicians, the American Thoracic Society, and SCCM.[8] Such groupings also launch joint projects, enable workgroups, and may host their own meetings. In general, participants in such ventures are drawn from the membership of the partnering organizations. Ninth, some medical professional organizations partner with international groups around specific initiatives, events, or clinical conditions. For example, SCCM and the European Society of Intensive Care Medicine has partnered to create the Surviving Sepsis Campaign, whose work is well known in a global fashion.[9] Participation in such related but more free-standing entities is not limited to membership in a parent organization but involved members who share work with experts from other organizations such as the Infectious Diseases Society of America,[10] or the American College of Emergency Physicians,[11] as well as the Japanese Association for Acute Medicine.[12] In summary, a wide array of networking, collaboration, and professional development benefits render the financial cost of membership well valued. These benefits are common across many organizations and are part of one's professional life and workflow. The recent severe acute respiratory syndrome coronavirus (SARS-CoV-2) pandemic has challenged medical professional organizations to respond in unique ways to support members in their pursuit of quality and timely clinical care. The ability of a given society to do so may hinge on the infrastructure that supports each of the above member benefits.

SARS-CoV-2 and medical professional organizations

As SARS-CoV-2 infection marched across continents, clinicians hungered for information encompassing all aspects of clinical care and public health. Diagnostic elements, infectivity risk, transmission pattern, clinical course, and evaluation of interventions—successful and not—were all highly desired. A country-by-country tally of those infected, recovered, and expired cases has emerged side by side with prediction models.[13] Contact tracing, social distancing, mask wearing, and hand hygiene permeated daily life.[14] Lockdowns, business closures, and household item shortages paralleled personal protective equipment shortages, as well as therapeutic agent shortages, in health-care facilities.[15] As life was put on hold, inquiries from professionals as well as the public blossomed. Social media (SoMe) exploded with myth, fears, tales of success, recounting of failure, and were interspersed with data, ever-changing recommendations, and despairingly little science. It is within this void that medical professional organizations rose to the fore to share information, credible new knowledge, and importantly, education for those who were not members of the organizations at all.

The process by which medical societies adapted to meet member and patients' needs may be conveniently grouped into nine interwoven domains (Fig. 3). Each of the domains leverage existing infrastructure including staff, technology, subject matter and content experts, as well as leadership within the organization, all of which is distinct from the volunteers to adapt to the imperatives launched by coronavirus disease 2019 (COVID-19) patient care. Importantly, such changes require a public-facing aspect so that members and nonmembers alike may be engaged in a seamless fashion. That public face is the website and webpage on which one lands when seeking to access content or learn about the organization.

Therefore website redesign is one key element undertaken by medical professional societies to readily direct website users to COVID-19 focused content. Tabs

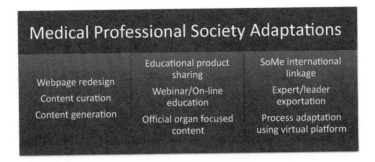

FIG. 3

Medical society roles.

or links rapidly appeared on the home page of multiple societies in response to member and nonmember searches. Of course, such direction must land the user on content. Content curation—from within and without the specific organization—became an essential task for staff, often requiring redeployment from prior projects or roles to dedicate sufficient time to identify, evaluate, and load appropriate content. This undertaking dovetailed with the third key society role—content development. As clinicians strove to decipher best practices, organizations rapidly generated both guidelines and guidance.

For example, the Surviving Sepsis Campaign, rapidly followed by the National Institutes of Health, each produced guidelines for immediate use in critical care areas from the Emergency Department to the intensive care unit (ICU).[16,17] More focused guidance around aerosol-generating procedures such as tracheostomy also followed from organizations such as the American College of Surgeons and the Surgical Infection Society.[18,19] Each of these documents helped clinicians decide on optimal care for those with SARS-CoV-2 infection.

As the volume of infected individuals skyrocketed, the need to understand resources, ICU capacity, and ideal methods of augmenting critical care spaces crested. Organizations such as SCCM crafted a key article as a blog post, not a journal article, that assessed resources and forecast where there may be shortages of devices and clinicians.[20] This pivot—from peer-reviewed manuscript to website blog post—signaled a shift to global knowledge dissemination in a move akin to that of Free Open Access Medical education and ensured that the content was not sheltered behind a paywall. As a follow-up, a second post assessed best practices for preparing ICU spaces and converting non-ICU spaces such as postanesthesia care unit rooms, general care floors, or conference halls into novel ICUs.[21] As space to provide critical care expanded, so too did the need for staff to competently work in those spaces. In this domain—clinician education—medical professional organizations excelled.

In parallel with posting resources on their websites, societies also released educational content that would help meet the need to enable non-ICU clinicians to render safe and effective care in the ICU. For example, SCCM's long-standing global product, the Fundamental Critical Care Support, teaches essential critical care skills to help rescue and provide the initial care for those with critical illness.[22] These resources were combined with others to create a program targeted at clinicians who would be redeployed to the ICU to help staff novel ICU spaces.[23] Importantly, these resources were made freely available as well, leading to widespread dissemination and use. Skills acquisition, new knowledge, or new perspectives on existing cognition are all supported in a team-based environment. Once such a new workforce is raised, it also benefits from leadership. Medical professional organizations also offer approaches to address leadership models for vastly expanded spaces. Tiered staffing strategies are particularly suited to utilize existing leaders as guides for new clinicians deployed to ICUs.[20] Those leaders include intensivists, nurse managers, bedside APPs, bedside critical care nurses, as well as ICU-focused PharmDs.

Web-based education occupies a foundational space in the overarching preparation of clinicians for COVID-19 patient care. Some elements develop so rapidly, raise controversy, or simply benefit from perspective sharing that another venue is required to keep clinicians up to date. Webinars meet this need. Multiple critical care focused societies, as well as those for whom critical care is part of their purview, hosted single society as well as joint society webinars joining experts with interested clinicians in a global fashion. Featured participants from different continents were readily linked on the participant's screen often without an access fee. Multiple formats spanning straightforward didactics to interactive debates punctuated daily workflow and liberally spilled over to weekend days as well. Commonly, webinars adopted a multiprofessional format appropriately mimicking the nature of ICU teams. Such ventures also joined organizations that had never previously worked together, or had not done so to elaborate educational materials. The success of these webinars drove some organizations to repeatedly partner event after event.

The professional medical journals working with, but not necessarily owned by medical professional organizations, also adapted to the hunger for information directly aligned with COVID-19 patient care. To wit, the *Journal of the American Medical Association* devoted specific content to a host of aspects of SARS-CoV-2-infected patient care including clinical data, perspectives, and research letters.[24] SCCM's *Critical Care Medicine*, *Pediatric Critical Care Medicine*, and *Critical Care Explorations* all offer focused direction to COVID-19-relevant articles for reader's ease of use.[25] Additionally, journals such as the *New England Journal of Medicine*, pushed COVID-19 content to interested readers.[26] Therefore the society's websites content and peer-reviewed journal content are all aligned to enhance clinical care and clinician knowledge.

Sharing new knowledge has been tremendously enabled by SoMe postings. Facebook and Twitter seem to dominate medically relevant information sharing compared to other platforms. Manuscripts published ahead of print, just-released press briefings from governmental agencies, and others are fired around the world, and shared repeatedly creating multiple digital echoes. Frequently, some posts are directed to a medical professional organization or to their official organ, toward a key leader, or a newly scheduled event. SoMe have helped craft a global critical care community during the pandemic with a previously unwitnessed intensity in the context of crisis care.[27]

Members and leaders of medical professional organizations were showcased on websites, webinars, and their messages were posted and published across multiple media platforms. This in turn supported such individuals to be recruited for multi-society ventures such as guidelines, virtual conferences, and in an unprecedented volume, media interview requests. Critical care medicine was catapulted into the headlines, the evening news, and opinion sections of newspapers. Relatedly, Merriam-Webster included "intensivist" as a new word this year during Critical Care Awareness month.[28] While key individuals were "exported" as experts, medical professional organizations also helped to "import" expert volunteer clinicians to sites needing staffing rescue. Organizations activated their member networks to secure volunteers to aid New York City, for example, leading to hundreds of clinicians from across the United States traveling to staff existing and novel ICUs. Many organizations around the globe have mechanisms to solicit volunteer aid during disasters including earthquakes, devastating hurricanes, floods, and pandemics. In this way, medical professional organizations support governmental relief and care efforts during disaster care—a key role that is easy to overlook—but which for the critically ill or injured may be lifesaving.

Throughout the pandemic, the business of medical societies and their volunteer activities needed to continue. Societies rapidly adopted virtual formats for committee work, leadership meetings, and collaboration with other organizations. For many clinicians, the platform used by the societies to which they belong was different from one another. Accordingly, members developed skill sets for using those platforms ahead of when virtual clinical care became feasible on a routine basis as part of a telemedicine approach to outpatient care. Platform competency also enabled many to use those skills to link patients, patient families, and the bedside care team in support of patient- and family-centered care while inhospital visitation was nearly entirely suspended.[29] Unwittingly, performing volunteer work for a medical professional society translated into prized inpatient and outpatient care skills.

Conclusion

Medical professional organizations can rapidly respond to member needs during a pandemic in support of education, information sharing, recommendations for clinical care, and upstaffing in response to a crisis. Their ability to do so leverages existing infrastructure and leadership, as well as a motivated and engaged volunteer member workforce to do so. In this process, members derive both personal and professional benefit while enhancing their ability to provide direct care. The impact of social media on each of these elements cannot be understated. It is likely that many of the adaptations medical professional organizations rapidly deployed in response to the SARS-CoV-2 pandemic will outlast the need for pandemic care.

References

1. American Board of Medical Specialties. https://www.abms.org/. Accessed 30 June 2020.
2. American Society of Anesthesiologists. https://www.asahq.org/. Accessed 30 June 2020.
3. Society of Critical Care Medicine. *SCCM | Society of Critical Care Medicine*. https://sccm.org/.
4. American Red Cross. https://www.redcross.org/. Accessed 30 June 2020.
5. Médecins Sans Frontières. https://www.msf.org/. Accessed 30 June 2020.
6. Centers for Disease Control and Prevention. https://www.cdc.gov/. Accessed 30 June 2020.
7. World Health Organization. *World Health Organization*. https://www.who.int/. Accessed 30 June 2020.
8. Critical Care Societies Collaborative. https://ccsconline.org/. Accessed 30 June 2020.
9. Rhodes A, Evans LE, Alhazzani W, et al. Surviving sepsis campaign: international guidelines for management of sepsis and septic shock: 2016. *Intensive Care Med.* 2017;43:304–377. https://doi.org/10.1007/s00134-017-4683-6.
10. Infectious Disease Society of America. https://www.idsociety.org/. Accessed 30 June 2020.
11. American College of Emergency Physicians. https://www.acep.org/. Accessed 30 June 2020.
12. Japanese Association for Acute Medicine. https://www.jaam.jp/english/english-top.html.
13. COVID-19 Dashboard by the Center for Systems Science and Engineering (CSSE) at Johns Hopkins University (JHU). https://gisanddata.maps.arcgis.com/apps/opsdashboard/index.html#/bda7594740fd40299423467b48e9ecf6. Accessed 3 July 2020.
14. Desai AN, Aronoff DM. Masks and coronavirus disease 2019 (COVID 19). *JAMA.* 2020;323(20):2103. https://doi.org/10.1001/jama.2020.6437.
15. Livingston E, Desai A, Berkwits M. Sourcing personal protective equipment during the COVID-19 pandemic. *JAMA.* 2020;323(19):1912–1914. https://doi.org/10.1001/jama.2020.5317.
16. Alhazzani W, Møller M, Arabi Y, et al. Surviving sepsis campaign: guidelines on the management of critically ill adults with coronavirus disease 2019 (COVID-19). *Intensive Care Med.* 2020;46(5):854–887. https://doi.org/10.1007/s00134-020-06022-5.
17. *NIH COVID-19 Treatment Guidelines*. https://www.covid19treatmentguidelines.nih.gov/. Accessed 30 June 2020.
18. *COVID-19: Considerations for Optimum Surgeon Protection Before, During, and After Operation*. American College of Surgeons; 2020. https://www.facs.org/covid-19/clinical-guidance/surgeon-protection. Accessed 30 June 2020.
19. Heffernan D, Evans H, Huston J, et al. Surgical infection society guidance for operative and peri-operative care of adult patients infected by the severe acute respiratory syndrome coronavirus-2 (SARS-CoV-2). *Surg Infect (Larchmt).* 2020;21(4):301–308. https://doi.org/10.1089/sur.2020.101.
20. Halpern N, Tan K. *United States Resource Availability for COVID-19*; 2020. March 13 https://sccm.org/Blog/March-2020/United-States-Resource-Availability-for-COVID-19. Accessed 30 June 2020.
21. Go KJ, Wong J, Tien JCC, et al. Preparing your intensive care unit for the COVID-19 pandemic: practical considerations and strategies. *Crit Care.* 2020;24:215.

22. Fundamental Critical Care Support. *Society of Critical Care Medicine*. https://www.sccm. org/Fundamentals/Fundamental-Critical-Care-Support. Accessed 30 June 2020.

23. Critical Care for Non-ICU Clinicians. https://www.sccm.org/Disaster/COVID19- ResourceResponseCenter. Accessed 3 July 2020.

24. Coronavirus (COVID19). *JAMA Network*. https://jamanetwork.com/collections/46099/ coronavirus-covid19. Accessed 30 June 2020.

25. *SCCM COVID-19 Journal Articles*. Society of Critical Care Medicine; 2020. https:// www.sccm.org/Member-Center/Journals/SCCM-COVID-19-Journal-Articles.

26. The New England Journal of Medicine Group. *COVID-19 Briefing*. https://www.nejm. org/coronavirus?query=main_nav_lg. Accessed 3 July 2020.

27. Chan AKM, Nickson CP, Rudolph JW, Lee A, Joynt GM. Social media for rapid knowledge dissemination: early experience from the COVID-19 pandemic. *Anaesthesia*. 2020. https://doi.org/10.1111/anae.15057.

28. Merriam-Webster. *We Added New Words to the Dictionary for April 2020*; 2020. https:// www.merriam-webster.com/words-at-play/new-words-in-the-dictionary. Accessed 30 June 2020.

29. Hart JL, Turnbull AE, Oppenheim IM, Courtright KR. Family-centered care during the COVID-19 era. *J Pain Symptom Manage*. 2020;60(2):e93–e97. https://doi.org/10.1016/ j.jpainsymman.2020.04.017.

Novel treatments and trials in COVID-19

10

Andrew Conway Morris[a,b] and Allison Tong[c]

[a]Division of Anaesthesia, Department of Medicine, University of Cambridge, Cambridge, United Kingdom, [b]John V Farm Intensive Care Unit, Addenbrooke's Hospital, Cambridge, United Kingdom, [c]Sydney School of Public Health, The University of Sydney, Sydney, NSW, Australia

Coronavirus disease 2019 (COVID-19), the disease arising from the beta coronavirus severe acute respiratory syndrome coronavirus 2 (SARS-CoV-2), has presented a major challenge to health-care systems and societies across the world.[1] Although previous highly pathogenic coronaviruses have emerged, namely severe acute respiratory syndrome coronavirus 1 (SARS-CoV-1) and Middle East respiratory syndrome coronavirus (MERS-CoV), neither had the spread nor the persistence to result in large clinical trials of drug therapy. Much of our therapeutic knowledge in these viruses was therefore informed by inference from observational, in vitro, and experimental model studies. As a result when SARS-CoV-2 emerged, with a noted high morbidity and mortality,[2] initial therapeutic drug treatment was often empiric.[2] There are currently over 4400 trials concerning COVID-19 registered on the World Health Organization international clinical trials registry, and while not all these are interventional therapeutic trials, this illustrates the desire of the international clinical-scientific community to develop systematic and evidence-based approaches for the management of this major threat.

This chapter discusses the broad strategies of therapeutic pharmacological approaches suggested, namely antiviral therapy, antiinflammatories, and immunomodulatory. Nonpharmacological approaches are also to be discussed. Then, it reviews the approaches to trials and trial design, the development and use of core outcome sets, and regulation of trials in pandemic settings. It reviews the publication and preprint availability of completed trials before discussing the ethics of empiric treatment outside the context of trials.

Therapeutic approaches

The three broad pharmacological approaches to COVID-19 are antiviral therapy, antiinflammatory, and immunomodulatory.

COVID-19 Pandemic. https://doi.org/10.1016/B978-0-323-82860-4.00006-9

Antivirals

COVID-19 arises from an interaction between the virus and the host immune response. Antiviral therapies have proven benefits in a range of viral infections, from human immunodeficiency virus (HIV) to hepatitis B and C and the Herpesviridae such as herpes simplex and cytomegalovirus.[3] The history of antiviral efficacy in respiratory viral illness is less positive, and while licensed treatments exist for influenza in the form of oseltamivir, its effect on illness course and mitigation of critical progression remain uncertain.[4] Evidence of effective antiviral therapy in SARS-CoV-1 and MERS-CoV-induced SARS was limited, with much of it coming from either animal models of disease or in vitro studies and no therapies proven in clinical trials.[5]

RNA-dependent RNA polymerase inhibitors

Originally developed for the treatment of the viral hemorrhagic fever Ebola arising from the filovirus *Zaire ebolavirus*, remdesivir is an RNA-dependent viral RNA polymerase inhibitor with broad in vitro activity against multiple families of viruses including Filoviridae, Pneumoviridae, and Orthocoronaviridae, the family to which the beta coronaviruses belong.[6] It had demonstrated efficacy in a mouse model of SARS-CoV-1 infection.[6] Recent trials in COVID-19 showed divergent outcomes, a study indicating faster resolution in hospitalized patients needing oxygen but not among those with more severe respiratory failure. However, the large SOLIDARITY trial did not demonstrate benefit.[7] Despite the negative results from the SOLIDARITY trial, Remdesivir retains emergency use authorization in a number of jurisdictions.

Favipiravir, which also targets RNA-dependent RNA polymerase, is being tested in number of ongoing trials, although completed studies to date are small, and efficacy remains to be proven.[8]

Protease inhibitors

Protease inhibitors are central to the management of HIV and also target proteases in Orthocoronaviridae.[5] In a marmoset model of MERS-CoV infection, the combination of lopinavir/ritonavir improved disease severity and viral clearance.[9] An early phase II randomized controlled trial comparing lopinavir/ritonavir with combination therapy, ribavirin and interferon beta suggested that combination therapy was superior to lopinavir/ritonavir alone.[10] However the lopinavir/ritonavir arms of the Randomized Evaluation of COVID-19 Therapy (RECOVERY) and SOLIDARITY trials indicate that it was not superior to placebo.[7,10,11]

Antimalarials

Chloroquine, and its derivative hydroxychloroquine, have well-established antimalarial activity. They are also commonly used in vitro for their effects on endosomal acidification and demonstrated in vitro activity against MERS-CoV.[12,13] Despite widespread adoption, concerns have been raised about the effect on cardiovascular mortality possibly linked to prolonged QT interval.[14] However, although neither the RECOVERY nor SOLIDARITY trials demonstrated any benefit of hydroxychloroquine,[7,15] they also did not indicate any excess of cardiovascular events attributed to this drug.

Antibiotics

Some antibacterial drugs also have antiviral properties, including azithromycin and teicoplanin.[16,17] Azithromycin has attracted particular attention as it may synergize with hydroxychloroquine, although the retrospective survey of patients reporting this has attracted notes of concern.[18,19]. The RECOVERY study azithromycin arm did not find any benefit, although neither did it find evidence of increased cardiac dysrhythmias.[20]

Convalescent plasma and immunoglobulins

Convalescent plasma, as a form of passive immunity, has a long history of use in viral illness, although large-scale randomized trials are lacking.[21] Convalescent plasma is a heterogenous treatment with varying titer levels, and although early use of high-titer plasma was associated with reduced disease progression in a small study of older adults,[22] the RECOVERY trial convalescent plasma arm was closed following a neutral result at interim analysis (formal publication is awaited). Although nonspecific intravenous immunoglobulin G is often used for patients with immunoglobulin G deficiencies for the prevention and treatment of infectious diseases, it also has immunosuppressive capabilities which are utilized in inflammatory diseases, specific evidence for its use in COVID-19 is lacking.

Antiinflammatories

Corticosteroids

Corticosteroids have long been used for ameliorating harmful inflammatory responses in infectious diseases, with proven roles in meningococcal septicemia and improvements in hemodynamics, and possibly mortality in septic shock.[23,24] Observational data suggested that their use may be harmful in MERS and SARS as well as pandemic influenza.[5,25] However, in COVID-19, several studies have demonstrated benefit among patients on mechanical ventilation or receiving oxygen, but not among the less severely unwell.[26]

Cytokine and complement blockade

Early observations that COVID-19 was associated with raised levels of cytokines, in common with other severe respiratory infections, have prompted interest in blockading proinflammatory cytokines.[27,28] Interleukin (IL)-6, for which there are several licensed biologic therapies, has been the dominant focus of therapeutic studies, with recent publications indicating efficacy in moderate to severe disease.[29] Additional therapies listed as being trialed on clinicaltrials.gov include blockade of complement C5 with ravulizumab, blockade of IL-1 with anakinra, tumor necrosis factor with infliximab, and colchicine as a broad-spectrum antiinflammatory, none of these trials have yet reported. An alternative approach targeting the intracellular signaling pathways such as the JAK-STAT pathway is also under investigation.

Immunomodulatory therapies

Although COVID-19, and indeed other severe infections, is associated with high levels of cytokinemia, there is evidence of secondary immune failure reflected in the high rate of secondary infections and impaired immune cells responses in the most severely unwell.[27,30] This has led to a number of ongoing trials of immunomodulatory drugs, including recombinant IL-7, granulocyte-macrophage colony-stimulating factor (GM-CSF), and blockade of the negative co-stimulatory molecule programmed cell death protein 1 with nivolumab. Interferon beta-1 has been trialed, usually in combination with protease inhibitors, following its efficacy in the marmoset model of MERS[10]; however, studies have not so far shown benefit.[7]

Mesenchymal stem cells (MSCs) have been trialed in acute respiratory distress syndrome (ARDS), and a small nonrandomized study was recently published in patients with COVID-19.[31,32] The mechanisms by which MSCs may improve outcomes are pluripotent but may include GM-CSF secretion, microvesicle release, enhanced fluid clearance, and pathogen phagocytosis.[33] The results of definitive treatment in COVID-19 are awaited.

Nonpharmacological interventions

For critically ill patients, many of the most well-proven interventions are nonpharmacological. Often these interventions seek to avoid harm caused by the organ support required for those with multiple organ failure and include low tidal ventilation and negative fluid balance in ARDS, restrictive transfusion thresholds, and late implementation of renal replacement therapy.[6,34–37] For patients with COVID-19 who meet the criteria for these previous trials, such interventions reflect best evidence-based supportive care. Proning of mechanically ventilated patients with ARDS is proven to improve mortality and demonstrates efficacy in COVID-19 as much as other causes of ARDS. Whether a similar approach is tolerable and effective in patients who do not require mechanical ventilation and sedation is being tested in several ongoing clinical trials, as are strategies for improving oxygenation and gas exchange such as noninvasive (mask) ventilation, high-flow nasal oxygen cannulae, and application of continuous positive airway pressure.

Timing of interventions

COVID-19 is a disease which starts with viral infection and progresses to an immunopathological state which may persist after the virus has been cleared and demonstrate discordance between presence of viral particles, inflammatory cell infiltration, and clinically apparent organ function.[38] It is likely that treatments that are effective at one stage of the disease may not be so effective at other stages. As an example, dexamethasone appears to be effective more than 7 days after the onset of symptoms, but not in the first 7 days while the apparent lack of efficacy of remdesivir among ventilated patients may reflect the relative late point at which ARDS develops relative to onset of symptoms.[26,27,39] While it remains speculative, it is possible that these differences reflect early viral proliferation that might be worsened by immunosuppressive corticosteroids, with later immunopathology that benefits.

Trial design

Clinical trials for novel therapeutics usually work their way through the widely adopted process of preclinical efficacy in cellular and animal models and toxicity testing before entering human studies. These then build through the phases from safety and dose finding (phase 1) usually undertaken in healthy volunteers, before early and midphase studies in the target patient population (phase 2) before entering the definitive phase 3 trials where clinical effectiveness in determining the outcomes of interest is tested. To get from a candidate molecule to licensed pharmaceutical can often take 10–15 years, and in a pandemic with urgent need for novel therapies, this timescale is clearly impractical. As a result, a number of processes have been adopted to try to reduce the time from discovery to implementation. As the proliferation of trials concerning COVID-19 has continued, repeated warnings have been issued about trial quality and rigor.[40]

Repurposing existing medication

As the review of therapeutic approaches above demonstrates, the dominant approach to treatment of COVID-19 is to repurpose existing pharmaceutical agents which are already licensed for alternative indications. Even where a drug has no existing license such as in the case of remdesivir, they were agents developed for other viral infections with at least preliminary use in humans. While this runs against the trend toward targeted drug design, it did allow early rapid implementation of phase 3 clinical trials.

Compassionate use and observational registry-based studies

When novel pathogens emerge, the lack of previous biological and clinical experience with them can make clinical decision making difficult. The imperative to try to treat and cure patients can then lead to empiric therapy, based on strategies derived

from similar diseases. During the COVID-19 pandemic, this was challenging as neither of the related diseases (MERS or SARS) has a strong underpinning of evidence.[5]
While the relationship between a single practitioner's individual therapeutic decisions and outcomes can never be determined with certainty, large-scale observational studies can allow detection of potential treatment effects but are at risk of
significant bias. As noted in the reviewed approaches above, several drugs that
had biologically plausible effects did not prove beneficial in phase 3 trials, and this
should sound a note of caution over the use of empiric therapy out-with the context of
a clinical trial.

Randomized controlled trials

Randomized controlled trials are the gold standard of clinical therapeutic investigations. While their use in the heterogenous syndromes that make up the dominant
workload in critical care has been questioned,[41] for well-defined disease states, they
remain our strongest defense against ineffective or dangerous interventions. There is
an extensive literature on the design, conduct, and evaluation of randomized trials,[42]
which are not reviewed in depth here, but key markers of trial quality have been identified and should be looked for when reviewing results. These refer not only to specific trial design features (randomization, blinding, handling of dropout, loss to
follow-up, a priori power calculations, and recruitment to power targets) but also
to trial conduct, which should include registration, publication of trial protocol
and statistical analysis plan prior to completion, and commitment to data availability
for post hoc analysis. Where trials are sponsored by commercial enterprises that may
benefit financially from the results, independence of the trial delivery, and analysis
team from that commercial entity should be looked for. Various investigator groups
have demonstrated that it is possible to deliver high-quality large randomized trials
despite the clinical and social pressures induced by the COVID-19 pandemic.

Complex innovative design

The desire to rapidly identify effective treatments for COVID-19 has led to more
widespread adoption of more complex and innovative trial designs.[43] Complex
innovative design (CID) covers a range of trial designs, including umbrella, multiarm, and adaptive approaches.[43] During the COVID-19 pandemic, platform trials,
which use combinations of multiarm and adaptive approaches underpinned by a
common protocol, have found favor. Notable examples of such approaches include
the RECOVERY, Randomized Embedded Multifactorial Adaptive Platform for
Community-acquired Pneumonia (REMAP-CAP),[5] and Solidarity platforms,
which have evaluated a range of interventions.[44–46] Through the use of common
control groups, against which each of the interventions can be assessed, and the
structured addition of intervention arms, these platforms can deliver rapid but

robustly evaluated results. REMAP-CAP is particularly interesting as it was a pre-existing adaptive study that was repurposed to include COVID-19. Adaptive trials allow for the conduct of the trial to be modified by the results it generates, and to include multiple and sometimes combined treatment arms.[47] This sort of design not only maximizes the efficiency of the study but also allows for examination of interactions between trial interventions.[47] CIDs need considerable thought and planning, and rapid implementation requires the infrastructure to be in place or able to be rapidly implemented. Funding foresight and investment in "potential trials" that are in place before they are needed are key to ensuring such studies can be successfully deployed.

Regulation of clinical trials

Clinical trials are conducted under the auspices of the national and local regulatory bodies, each of which has its own requirements and procedures. The international committee on harmonization has sought to establish common standards across many of the major regions conducting clinical trials, ensuring that results from one region can be used for regulatory approvals in another. In the context of a rapidly evolving global pandemic, this becomes increasingly important.

Core outcomes

There has been a proliferation of trials in response to COVID-19, however, the wide heterogeneity of outcomes reported and omission of patient-reported outcomes can limit the use of this evidence for informed decision making. Core outcome sets can improve consistency in the reporting of critically important outcomes. Four initiatives have been established for COVID-19, and all have identified mortality and respiratory failure as core outcomes.[48–52] The World Health Organization candidate core outcome measure sets include viral burden, survival, and clinical progression to assess the severity of disease.[48] Recently, the global COVID-19 Core Outcomes Set initiative was launched to establish core outcomes for people with suspected or confirmed COVID-19. Based on a systematic review of outcomes reported, published and registered trials, an international online survey conducted in five languages involving 9289 patients, caregivers, health professionals and members of the general public from 111 countries, and four consensus workshops, five core outcome domains were identified: mortality, respiratory failure, multiorgan failure, shortness of breath, and recovery[51,52] and the core outcome measures arising from these have been published.[53] The implementation of core outcomes in trials in COVID-19 can help to ensure that outcomes of critical importance to all stakeholders are consistently reported in trials to better support informed decision making.

Publication and preprints

COVID-19 has seen an explosion in the use of clinical study and trial preprints, where manuscripts are posted on a publicly available server prior to peer review. The major medical and biological preprint servers, MedRxiv and BioRxiv, currently record 5230 and 1345 COVID-19 manuscripts, respectively. In contrast, MedRxiv records only 2355 manuscripts concerning influenza, a far more long-standing viral threat. The advantage of preprint deposition is that it allows for rapid dissemination of key findings, which during a fast-moving pandemic can help inform clinical decision making. However, as preprints will only have been reviewed within the research team, there is a greater potential for flawed or incomplete results to be released, and readers will have to conduct a higher degree of critical appraisal themselves. However, it also allows for "community peer review," which was perhaps most clearly seen following the release of the dexamethasone arm of the recovery trial.[54] Preprints do not replace formal peer-reviewed publication but should be seen as rapid notification of preliminary results.

Ethics of empiric therapy outside clinical trials

At the core of medical ethics lie the principles of autonomy (allowing the patient to make informed decisions), nonmaleficence (first do not harm), beneficence (serving the best interests of the patient), and justice (ensuring equitable treatment to all patients). While the treatment imperative may seem to demand action, one of the key lessons from the experience of COVID-19 has been of the perils of empiric therapy founded on personal clinical experience and biologically plausible therapies not subjected to clinical testing. These may violate several principles of medical ethics, as patients may come to harm with no potential for benefit, while being denied both the personal and wider societal benefits that may accrue from participation in clinical trials. Patients should be offered the best-proven treatments, including supportive care. Where empirical therapies are considered, these are the most ethically delivered in the context of an appropriately designed and regulated clinical trial. Where this is not possible, consenting patient data should be submitted to case registries.

In conclusion, COVID-19 has presented a major challenge to health-care services as clinicians have urgently sought effective treatments. Reliance of limited experience from previous similar diseases sometimes led to the use of empiric therapies which, when tested in large randomized trials, prove to be ineffective. As it has been possible to deliver high-quality, multicenter, and indeed multinational trials during the pandemic, this approach is likely to improve outcomes for patients with COVID-19.

References

1. Dong E, Du H, Gardner L. An interactive web-based dashboard to track COVID-19 in real time. *Lancet Infect Dis.* 2020;20(5):533–534.
2. Chen N, Zhou M, Dong X, et al. Epidemiological and clinical characteristics of 99 cases of 2019 novel coronavirus pneumonia in Wuhan, China: a descriptive study. *Lancet.* 2020;395:507–513.
3. De Clercq E, Li G. Approved antiviral drugs over the past 50 years. *Clin Microbiol Rev.* 2016;29:695–747.
4. Heneghan CJ, Onakpoya I, Jones MA, et al. Neuraminidase inhibitors for influenza: a systematic review and meta-analysis of regulatory and mortality data. *Health Technol Assess.* 2016;20:1–242.
5. Zumla A, Chan JFW, Azhar EI, Hui DSC, Yuen K-Y. Coronaviruses – drug discovery and therapeutic options. *Nat Rev Drug Discov.* 2016;15:327–347.
6. Sheahan TP, Sims AC, Graham RL, et al. Broad-spectrum antiviral GS-5734 inhibits both epidemic and zoonotic coronaviruses. *Sci Trans Med.* 2017;9. eaal3653–20.
7. Pan H, Peto R, et al, WHO Solidarity Trial Consortium. Repurposed antiviral drugs for Covid-19—interim WHO solidarity trial results. *N Engl J Med.* 2021;384:497–511.
8. Shiraki K, Daikoku T. Favipiravir, an anti-influenza drug against life-threatening RNA virus infections. *Pharmacol Ther.* 2020;209:107512–107516.
9. Chan JF-W, Yao Y, Yeung M-L, et al. Treatment with lopinavir/ritonavir or interferon-β 1b improves outcome of MERS-CoV infection in a non-human primate model of common marmoset. *J Infect Dis.* 2015;212:1904–1913.
10. Hung IF-N, Lung K-C, Tso EY-K, et al. Triple combination of interferon beta-1b, lopinavir-ritonavir, and ribavirin in the treatment of patients admitted to hospital with COVID-19: an open-label, randomised, phase 2 trial. *Lancet.* 2020;395:1695–1704.
11. RECOVERY Collaborative Group. Lopinavir-ritonavir in patients admitted to hospital with COVID-19 (RECOVERY): a randomised, controlled, open-label, platform trial. *Lancet.* 2020;396(10259):1345–1352.
12. Al-Bari MAA. Targeting endosomal acidification by chloroquine analogs as a promising strategy for the treatment of emerging viral diseases. *Pharmacol Res Perspect.* 2017;5: e00293.
13. de Wilde AH, Jochmans D, Posthuma CC, et al. Screening of an FDA-approved compound library identifies four small-molecule inhibitors of Middle East respiratory syndrome coronavirus replication in cell culture. *Antimicrob Agents Chemother.* 2014;58:4875–4884.
14. Jankelson L, Karam G, Becker ML, Chinitz LA, Tsai M-C. QT prolongation, torsades de pointes, and sudden death with short courses of chloroquine or hydroxychloroquine as used in COVID-19: a systematic review. *Heart Rhythm.* 2020;17(9):1472–1479.
15. Horby P, Mafham M, Linsell L, RECOVERY Collaborative Group, et al. Effect of hydroxychloroquine in hospitalized patients with COVID-19: preliminary results from a multicentre, randomized, controlled trial. *New Eng J Med.* 2020;383:2030–2040. https://doi. org/10.1101/2020.07.15.20151852.
16. Madrid PB, Panchal RG, Warren TK, et al. Evaluation of Ebola virus inhibitors for drug repurposing. *ACS Infect Dis.* 2015;1:317–326.

17. Wang Y, Cui R, Li G, et al. Teicoplanin inhibits Ebola pseudovirus infection in cell culture. *Antiviral Res.* 2016;125:1–7.

18. Gautret P, Lagier J-C, Parola P, et al. Hydroxychloroquine and azithromycin as a treatment of COVID-19: results of an open-label non-randomized clinical trial. *Int J Antimicrob Agents.* 2020;56:105949.

19. Official Statement from International Society of Antimicrobial Chemotherapy (ISAC). *Hydroxychloroquine and azithromycin as a treatment of COVID-19: results of an open-label non-randomized clinical trial (Gautret P et al. PMID 32205204);* 2020. https://www.isac.world/news-and-publications/official-isac-statement.

20. Horby PJ, RECOVERY Collaborative Group, et al. Azithromycin in patients admitted to hospital with COVID-19 (RECOVERY): a randomised, controlled, open-label, platform trial. *Lancet.* 2021;397:605–612.

21. Marano G, Vaglio S, Pupella S, et al. Convalescent plasma: new evidence for an old therapeutic tool? *Blood Transfus.* 2016;14:152–157.

22. Libster R, Pérez Marc G, Wappner D, Fundación INFANT–COVID-19 Group, et al. Early high-titer plasma therapy to prevent severe Covid-19 in older adults. *N Eng J Med.* 2021;384:610–618.

23. Brouwer MC, McIntyre P, Prasad K, van de Beek D. Corticosteroids for acute bacterial meningitis. Cochrane Acute Respiratory Infections Group, ed. *Cochrane Database Syst Rev.* 2015;31:53–86.

24. Annane D, Bellissant E, Bollaert P-E, et al. Corticosteroids for treating sepsis in children and adults. Cochrane Emergency and Critical Care Group, ed. *Cochrane Database Syst Rev.* 2019;12:CD002243.

25. Zhang Y, Sun W, Svendsen ER, et al. Do corticosteroids reduce the mortality of influenza A (H1N1) infection? A meta-analysis. *Crit Care.* 2015;19:46.

26. Sterne JAC, Murthy S, Diaz JV, WHO Rapid Evidence Appraisal for COVID-19 Therapies (REACT) Working Group, et al. Association between administration of systemic corticosteroids and mortality among critically ill patients with COVID-19: a meta-analysis. *JAMA.* 2020;324:1330–1341.

27. Zhou F, Yu T, Du R, et al. Clinical course and risk factors for mortality of adult inpatients with COVID-19 in Wuhan, China: a retrospective cohort study. *Lancet.* 2020;395 (10229):1054–1062.

28. Conway Morris A, Kefala K, Wilkinson TS, et al. Diagnostic importance of pulmonary interleukin-1 and interleukin-8 in ventilator-associated pneumonia. *Thorax.* 2010;65: 201–207.

29. Gordon AC, Mouncey PR, Al-Beidh F, REMAP-CAP Investigators, et al. Interleukin-6 receptor antagonists in critically ill patients with Covid-19. *N Eng J Med.* 2021. https://doi.org/10.1056/NEJMoa2100433, PMC7953461.

30. Jeannet R, Daix T, Formento R, Feuillard J, François B. Severe COVID-19 is associated with deep and sustained multifaceted cellular immunosuppression. *Intensive Care Med.* 2020;46:1769–1771.

31. Matthay MA, Calfee CS, Zhuo H, et al. Treatment with allogeneic mesenchymal stromal cells for moderate to severe acute respiratory distress syndrome (START study): a randomised phase 2a safety trial. *Lancet Resp Med.* 2019;7(2):154–162.

32. Leng Z, Zhu R, Hou W, et al. Transplantation of ACE2- mesenchymal stem cells improves the outcome of patients with COVID-19 pneumonia. *Aging Dis.* 2020;11:216–228.

33. Laffey JG, Matthay MA. Fifty years of research in ARDS. Cell-based therapy for acute respiratory distress syndrome. Biology and potential therapeutic value. *Am J Respir Crit Care Med.* 2017;196:266–273.
34. ARDSnet. Ventilation with lower tidal volumes as compared with traditional tidal volumes for acute lung injury and the acute respiratory distress syndrome. The Acute Respiratory Distress Syndrome Network. *N Engl J Med.* 2000;342:1301–1308.
35. National Heart, Lung, and Blood Institute Acute Respiratory Distress Syndrome (ARDS) Clinical Trials Network, Wiedemann HP, Wheeler AP, et al. Comparison of two fluid-management strategies in acute lung injury. *N Engl J Med.* 2006;354:2564–2575.
36. Hébert PC, Wells G, Blajchman MA, et al. A multicenter, randomized, controlled clinical trial of transfusion requirements in critical care. *N Engl J Med.* 1999;340:409–417.
37. Gaudry S, Hajage D, Benichou N, et al. Delayed versus early initiation of renal replacement therapy for severe acute kidney injury: a systematic review and individual patient data meta-analysis of randomised clinical trials. *Lancet.* 2020;395:1506–1515.
38. Dorward DA, Russell CD, Um IH, Elshani M. Tissue-specific tolerance in fatal Covid-19. *MedRxivorg.* 2020. https://doi.org/10.1101/2020.07.02.20145003.
39. Beigel JH, Tomashek KM, Dodd LE. Remdesivir for the treatment of covid-19—preliminary report. *New Eng J Med.* 2020;383:1813–1826.
40. Bonini S, Maltese G. COVID-19 clinical trials: quality matters more than quantity. *Allergy.* 2020;2(6):e286.
41. Ospina-Tascón GA, Büchele GL, Vincent J-L. Multicenter, randomized, controlled trials evaluating mortality in intensive care: doomed to fail? *Crit Care Med.* 2008;36:1311–1322.
42. Berger VW, Alperson SY. A general framework for the evaluation of clinical trial quality. *Rev Recent Clin Trials.* 2009;4:79–88.
43. Navie W. *The rise of Complex Innovative Design (CID) trials during the COVID-19 pandemic*; 2020. https://www.hra.nhs.uk/about-us/news-updates/rise-complex-innovative-design-cid-trials-during-covid-19-pandemic-blog-hra-engagement-manager-will-navaie/. Accessed 15 July 2020.
44. RECOVERY trial. https://www.recoverytrial.net. Accessed 15 July 2020.
45. REMAP-CAP trial. https://www.remapcap.org. Accessed 15 July 2020.
46. Solidarity trial. https://www.who.int/emergencies/diseases/novel-coronavirus-2019/global-research-on-novel-coronavirus-2019-ncov/solidarity-clinical-trial-for-covid-19-treatments. Accessed 15 July 2020.
47. Curtin F, Heritier S. The role of adaptive trial designs in drug development. *Expert Rev Clin Pharm.* 2017;10:727–736.
48. Marshall JC, Murthy S, Diaz J, et al. A minimal common outcome measure set for COVID-19 clinical research. *Lancet Infect Dis.* 2020;1–6.
49. Jin X, Pang B, Zhang J, et al. Core outcome set for clinical trials on coronavirus disease 2019 (COS-COVID). *Engineering (Beijing).* 2020;6:1147–1152.
50. *Core outcome set developers' response to COVID-19 (7th July 2020)*; 2020. http://www.comet-initiative.org/Studies/Details/1538. Accessed 16 July 2020.
51. Tong A, Elliott JH, Cesar Azevedo L, et al. Core outcomes set for people with COVID-19. *Crit Care Med.* 2020;48:1622–1635.
52. Evangelidis N, Tong A, Howell M, et al. International survey to establish prioritized outcomes for trials in people with COVID-19. *Crit Care Med.* 2020;48:1612–1621.

53. Tong A, Elliott JH, Azevedo LC, COVID-19-Core Outcomes Set (COS) Workshop Investigators, et al. Core outcomes set for trials in people with coronavirus disease 2019. *Crit Care Med*. 2020;48:1622–1635.

54. Neporent L. *Coronavirus Social: Twitter's Mixed Response to Dexamethasone Preprint*. Medscape.com; 2020. https://www.medscape.com/viewarticle/933012?nlid=136105_5170&src=WNL_ukmdpls_200627_mscpedit_gen&uac=32560SY&impID=2437228&faf=1. Accessed 15 July 2020.

COVID-19: Lessons from the frontline

11

Natalia Largaespada Beer and Lorna Pérez

Ministry of Health, Belmopan, Belize

Background

The global spread of coronavirus disease 2019 (COVID-19) within a 12-week period had countries globally grappling to meet the demands of the unknowns of this pandemic. Health-care systems have been reeling with demands placing it in a critical state to meet the needs of the population.[a] As of August 6, 2020, 18.8 million cases of COVID-19 have been diagnosed worldwide of which 11.3 million (60.1%) have recovered and 706,000 deaths occurred, with 216 countries reporting active cases. The countries reporting more than 1 million confirmed cases are United States, Brazil, and India. The United States exhibits the lowest proportion of recovered patients (49.4%) compared to Brazil and India, each with 70% of confirmed cases recovered. India has the lowest percentage of confirmed cases who died (2.1%).

On January 10, the World Health Organization (WHO) issued an advisory to all nations to prepare for a novel virus now known as severe acute respiratory syndrome coronavirus 2 (SARS-CoV-2) causing severe respiratory disease, which had been reported in Wuhan, China in December 2019. The call was for countries to revise their influenza plans and identify gaps, conduct risk assessments, and plan for investigation, prevention, and response in the event the country experiences an outbreak. On January 30, the WHO declared the COVID-19 outbreak a public health emergency of international concern meaning that there was the potential of global transmission of the virus. On March 11, the WHO declared COVID-19 a pandemic as COVID-19 was being reported by almost all countries.

Introduction

The WHO defines a pandemic as the worldwide spread of a new disease. In this case, a novel SARS-CoV emerged in Wuhan, China, and spreads around the world in less than 3 months, and most people do not have immunity. With the advances in information technology and research capacity, the global scientific community has

---

[a]https:/covid19.who.int/ Accessed: June 1, 2020, 14:08 hours

COVID-19 Pandemic. https://doi.org/10.1016/B978-0-323-82860-4.00005-7

invested efforts to obtain data on the SARS-CoV-2 virus to aid countries in their preparation and response to the pandemic. In recent years, the WHO has prompted countries to develop and implement their national influenza preparedness plans, and this has helped countries to fast track their response plan to the 2019 novel SARS-CoV-2 disease or COVID-19 pandemic.

National Response Plan to COVID-19 pandemic

Similarly, to the pandemic influenza plans, a comprehensive national response plan contains the following technical areas:[b]

- oversight of the national response
- assessment of the readiness of the health system
- surveillance, epidemiology, and laboratory activities[2]
- community empowerment and mitigation measures
- medical equipment and supplies for patient care
- infection prevention and control
- Clinical guidelines
- Risk communication plan

The national response to the COVID-19 pandemic and the learning of the characteristics of the 2019 novel SARS-CoV-2 demanded from countries to strengthen their multisectoral response and to use the rapidly changing evidence to make decisions and for the national and subnational response teams to be open to overwhelming flexibility in the response.

The national response to COVID-19, a national challenge

This section offers practical recommendations of each of the technical areas enlisted in the "Introduction" section.

National oversight committee

Countries learnt on the go that the impact of the COVID-19 pandemic is way beyond the health sector. Every citizen is affected by the consequences of the pandemic, especially in the economic sphere as some drastic lifesaving measures ought to be put in place to contain and mitigate the increase in morbidity and mortality; hence, the need to have a national oversight committee who is responsible for the multisector response to the pandemic. This committee is chaired by the highest governmental authorities from key sectors such as national security, economic development, human development, health and education, and ministry of finance. The decisions made at that level are then communicated to the population. Frequent press

---

[b]U.S. Department of Health and Human Services. Pandemic influenza plan. 2017 Update.

conferences allow the media and the population through social media to voice their concerns and to be offered an explanation to each of their questions. The committee meets on a weekly basis or as often needed.

The COVID-19 pandemic impels governments through their national oversight committees to take drastic measures as per legislative prerogatives. They are not known to be friendly, rather they are measures to contribute to the preservation of life. Examples of drastic measures that have short-, medium-, and long-term effects are Declaration of State of Emergency, curfew, closing of schools, closing of the borders, quarantined communities with high number of cases, and restriction of movement within and across districts.

Assessment of the readiness of the health system

The COVID-19 causes an upper respiratory infection that progresses to a systemic illness and eventually death for those who have negative risk factors. The following documents are available to help countries to assess their health system readiness and technical guides for preparation of the national response to COVID-19: reagent calculator (August 3, 2020), guidance for conducting a country COVID-19 intra-action review (July 23, 2020), practical actions in cities to strengthen preparedness for the COVID-19 pandemic and beyond (July 17, 2020), investing in and building long-term health emergency preparedness during the COVID-19 pandemic (July 6, 2020), monitoring and evaluation plan (June 5, 2020), operational planning guidance to support country preparedness and response (May 22, 2020), strategic preparedness and response plan (April 14, 2020); assessment tool for laboratories implementing COVID-19 virus testing: interim guidance (April 8, 2020), national capacities review tool for a novel coronavirus (January 9, 2020), and preparing for a large-scale community transmission of COVID-19 (February 28, 2020), among others. The systematic assessment of the readiness of the health system allows for early identification of needs and actions to close the gaps in an orderly and phased manner, from most to less critical gaps. The systematic assessment allows for the documentation of the process followed in preparing the health system for an effective response.

National COVID-19 surveillance system

The WHO prepared and shared the case definitions of COVID-19 since January 11, 2020 which was updated four times. The last update was August 7, 2020 (Figs. 1 and 2). It can be found at: https:/www.who.int/publications/i/item/WHO-2019-nCoV-Surveillance_Case_Definition-2020.1

The surveillance system for COVID-19 should be geographically comprehensive and includes all persons and communities at risk, combined across different sites to collect data comprehensively. The objective of the COVID-19 surveillance is to enable rapid detection, isolation, testing, and management of suspected cases; guide the implementation of control measures; detect and contain outbreaks among vulnerable populations; evaluate the impact of the pandemic on the health-care system and

Case definition (Jan 28, 2020)   **Case Definition (Mar 20, 2020)**

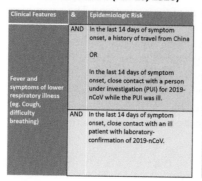

Clinical Features	&	Epidemiologic Risk
Fever and symptoms of lower respiratory illness (eg. Cough, difficulty breathing)	AND	In the last 14 days of symptom onset, a history of travel from China OR In the last 14 days of symptom onset, close contact with a person under investigation (PUI) for 2019-nCoV while the PUI was ill.
	AND	In the last 14 days of symptom onset, close contact with an ill patient with laboratory-confirmation of 2019-nCoV.

A. A patient with acute respiratory illness (fever and at least one sign/symptom of respiratory disease, e.g., cough, shortness of breath), AND a history of travel to or residence in a location reporting community transmission of COVID-19 disease during the 14 days prior to symptom onset; OR

B. A patient with any acute respiratory illness AND having been in contact with a confirmed or probable COVID-19 case (see definition of contact) in the last 14 days prior to symptom onset; OR

C. A patient with severe acute respiratory illness (fever and at least one sign/symptom of respiratory disease, e.g., cough, shortness of breath; AND requiring hospitalization) AND in the absence of an alternative diagnosis that fully explains the clinical presentation.

FIG. 1

COVID-19 case definitions 1 and 2.

Case definition (August 7, 2020)

Suspected case	Probable case	Confirmed case
Clinical criteria Acute onset of fever AND cough Or any three or more: fever, cough, general weakness/fatigue, headache, myalgia, sore throat, dyspnea, anorexia/nausea/vomiting, diarrhea, altered mental status AND Residing or working in an rea with high risk transmission of the virus **Or epidemiological criteria** Reside or travel to areas with community transmission within 14 days prior to the onset of symptoms Or Working in health care setting A patient with severe acute respiratory illness	A patient who meets clinical criteria and is a contact of a confirmed case or epidemiologically linked to a cluster with at least one confirmed case, or Suspect case with chest imaging suggestive of COVID-19 disease A person with recent anosmia (loss of smell) or ageusia (loss of taste) in the absence of any other identified cause, or Death not otherwise explained, in an adult with respiratory distress preceding death and was a contact of a probable or confirmed case or epidemiologically linked to a cluster with at least one confirmed case	A person with laboratory confirmation of COVID-19 infection, irrespective of clinical signs and symptoms.

FIG. 2

COVID-19 case definition 3.

Source: Epidemiology Unit, Ministry of Health, Belize.

society; monitor long-term epidemiologic trends and evolution of COVID-19 virus; and understand the co-circulation of COVID-19 virus, influenza, and other respiratory viruses. Table 1 outlines the combination of type of surveillance with surveillance sites, which serves as a guide to countries.[c]

The COVID-19 surveillance system is the cornerstone for the containment and mitigation of COVID-19 pandemic. For it to be effective, all other technical areas are required, for example, risk communication, laboratory services, human resources for health, enhanced infection prevention and control, among others.

The generic contacts risk classification shared by the global public health specialists needs to be tailored to the country's context. The risk classification is a group of standards to aid the frontline workers to make decisions regarding the case management. It also contributes to the effective use of resources and effective active search for potential cases. Table 2 shows the contacts risk classification used in Belize.

The contact tracing allows the epidemiological surveillance teams to identify cases and their contacts to halt the transmission of the virus at community level, workstations, and other settings. It allows for indirect measurement of compliance with recommended public health measures. Fig. 3 depicts the number of cases and the number of identified contacts of each case in a small group of infected persons.

Preparatory works to face the COVID-19 pandemic must include the ports of entry. Knowing who enters a country, their whereabouts, and determining their status will facilitate the tracking of persons under investigation or persons with a confirmed SARS-CoV-2 diagnosis. All employees coming in contact with persons entering the country (Immigration and Customs) must be knowledgeable of the process to follow for the receipt and screening and the case management of their nationals, residents, and tourists. A plan must be in place to track their movement within the country for at least 14 days or more if positive until recovery. The port of entry staff must be trained on how to use the different forms of documentation (application, tablet, software, or hard copy). All these must have a written process to be shared and standardized among staff. Table 3 shows the port of entry activities during 60 days prior to the closing of the borders.

The globally recommended public health measures must be tailored to the local context. They include, for example, frequent handwashing, physical distance of minimum 6 feet, staying at home or lockdown, cough etiquette and proper use of face mask, covering nose and chin, among others. For pregnant women, the two additional measures are stay away from sick people and avoid unnecessary exposure to crowded places, e.g., supermarket (Fig. 4). Pregnant women with COVID-19 have double and triple risk for coagulopathies of obstetric or infectious origin.

---

[c]WHO. Surveillance strategies for COVID-19 human infection. Coronavirus (COVID-19) update No. 29, June 5, 2020.

Table 1 Type of surveillance and surveillance sites.

Type of surveillance	Surveillance sites					
	Individuals in the community	Primary care sites (non-sentinel ILI/SARI)	Hospitals (non-sentinel ILI/SARI)	Sentinel ILI/SARI	Residential facilities and vulnerable groups	Vital statistics office
Immediate case notification system	×	×	×	×	×	
Contact tracing system	×					
Sentinel virus surveillance			×	×		
Sentinel case surveillance			×	×		
Cluster investigations	×	×	×	×		
Special settings			×		×	
Mortality	×		×	×	×	×

Source: Epidemiology Unit, Ministry of Health, Belize.

Table 2 COVID-19 risk classification.

High-risk contacts
- Living in the same household as, being an intimate partner of, or providing care in a non-health-care setting (such as a home) for a person with symptomatic laboratory-confirmed 2019 novel coronavirus infection "without using recommended precautions" for home care and home isolation.
- The same risk assessment applies for the above-listed exposures to a person diagnosed clinically with COVID-19 infection outside of Belize who did not have laboratory testing.

Medium-risk contacts
- Close contact with a person diagnosed clinically with symptomatic laboratory-confirmed COVID-19 infection, and not having any exposures that meet a high-risk definition.
  ○ This also applies for close contact with a person diagnosed clinically with COVID-19 infection outside of Belize who did not have laboratory testing.
  ○ On an aircraft, being seated within 6 feet (2 meters) of a traveler with symptomatic laboratory-confirmed COVID-19 infection; this distance correlates approximately with two seats in each direction.
- Living in the same household as, being an intimate partner of, or providing care in a non-health-care setting (such as a home) for a person with symptomatic laboratory-confirmed COVID-19 infection "while consistently using recommended precautions" for home care and home isolation.
- Travel from countries with active transmission AND not having any exposures that meet a high-risk definition.

Low-risk contacts
- Being in the same indoor environment (e.g., a classroom, a hospital waiting room) as a person with symptomatic laboratory-confirmed COVID-19 infection for a prolonged period of time but not meeting the definition of close contact.
- On an aircraft, being seated within two rows of a traveler with symptomatic laboratory-confirmed COVID-19 infection but not within 6 feet (2 m) AND not having any exposures that meet a medium- or a high-risk definition.

No identifiable risk
- Interactions with a person clinically diagnosed with symptomatic laboratory-confirmed COVID-19 infection that do not meet any of the high-, medium-, or low-risk conditions above, such as walking by the person or being briefly in the same room.

Source: Epidemiology Unit, Ministry of Health, Belize.

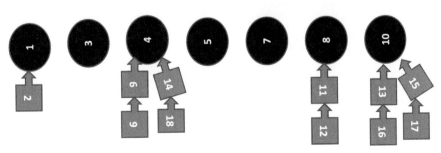

FIG. 3

COVID-19 positive cases, in chronological order, Belize, March—April, 2020.

Source: Epidemiology Unit, Ministry of Health, Belize

Table 3 Summary of screening at the port of entry.

• Highest number/day	2500
• Total vessels	1229
• Total passengers and crew	104,048
• Cruise passenger arrivals	359,743

Source: Epidemiology Unit, Ministry of Health, Belize.

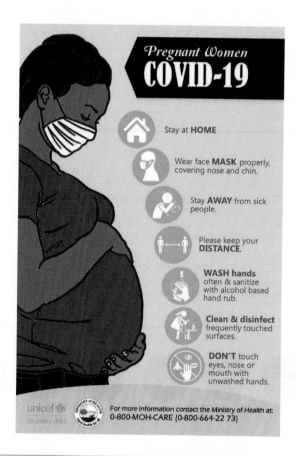

FIG. 4

Transmission precaution measures—pregnancy.

Source: HECOPAB, Ministry of Health, Belize.

COVID-19 epidemiology

Epidemiology is the use of data collected in a systematic manner to study the distribution and determinants of health-related states or events in specified populations and its application to control health problems.[d] In the mid-1980s, five major tasks of epidemiology in public health practice were identified: public health surveillance, field investigation, analytic studies, evaluation, and linkages.[e] Until recently, policy development is considered a task of epidemiology in public health. The demand from country's epidemiology units in the COVID-19 pandemic surpasses the national capacity as gaps in human resources also affects nonclinical units. COVID-19 demands a greater presence of experts in epidemiology in the field to aid with the local response based on data analysis.

Laboratory services

The 2019 novel SARS-CoV-2 virus caught many low- and middle-income countries (LMIC) off guard, as the gold standard test recommended for diagnosis of the virus, Reverse transcription polymerase chain reaction may have not been available before the declaration of the pandemic. LMIC countries usually build their laboratory capacity as a result of project or study opportunities which include hardware equipment. The laboratory services are one of the first to be fully equipped by any means with human resource, hardware, software, medical supplies, and updated guidelines for the early detection of cases. There are many other types of antibody testing for COVID-19 of which many are still in validation process. Having access to automated laboratory equipment have facilitated the timeliness and accuracy of results by reducing the potential for human error during the process of diagnosis. The use of antibody tests that are not safe and can lead to undesirable outcomes and unnecessary exposure of limited health professionals.

Community empowerment and mitigation measures

Informed and empowered communities can effectively contribute to the containment and mitigation of COVID-19. Because of the alarming speed of the pandemic and the access to social media of the effects of COVID-19 in developing countries, less developed countries because of the predominance of negative social determinants of health, the public health measures to contain the virus were not easily accepted and practiced. When the public health measures are overlapping with basic human rights, the compliance with transmission prevention measures becomes difficult.

[d]Last JM, editor. Dictionary of epidemiology. 4th ed. New York: Oxford University Press; 2001. p. 61.
[e]Tyler CW, Last JM. Epidemiology. In: Last JM, Wallace RB, editors. Maxcy-Rosenau-Last public health and preventive medicine, 14th ed. Norwalk (Connecticut): Appleton & Lange; 1992. p. 11.

Medical equipment and supplies for patient care

The novel coronavirus 2019 or SARS-CoV-2, is here to stay. The medical equipment and medical supplies required for the provision of patient care can be secured through large investments (new health infrastructures), projects (enhancing existing services) or for small countries utilizing existing resources to reorganize the services provided to the population. Each country faces the challenge of decision making based on epidemiological models that projects the estimated total number of cases and those requiring hospital or inpatient services.

Similar analysis needs to be done for the decision making on human resources for health (HRH) to face the response to COVID-19. Are there resources to increase the HRH? Or the health system needs to be reorganized for the existing HRH to provide services to those affected by COVID-19? Or the epidemiological surveillance response is effective enough to contain the spread of the disease by giving priority to the prevention and mitigation measures at community level for early identification and follow up of suspicious and confirmed cases? This requires a honest review of the HRH at all levels of care.

Infection prevention and control

Infection and prevention control (IPC) measures are pivotal to the prevention and control of the spread of the SARS-CoV-2 virus that causes COVID-19. The global pandemic reminds us of the importance of IPC measures to prevent or control transmissible diseases. The IPC measures are applicable to health facilities, homes, and institutions of all types. The global pandemic highlighted the need for strong investment and updating of IPC measures to stop the transmission of the virus in all spheres. Implementing the IPC measures in business settings, the willingness and creativity of business owners to protect their consumers, their workers, and the community at large is commendable. IPC is an area that received collaboration from the private sector for activities implemented at local health facilities and communities. Although the creativity was enhanced, the new normal is challenging the behavior from individuals and families. There are success stories of clusters of families who did not infect any other individuals. On the other hand, there are far more stories of persons who tested positive and find creative ways to breach the recommended and regulated quarantine or home isolation periods, transmitting the virus to others.

Clinical guidelines

The global pandemic leads rapidly to the massive sharing of information to improve the quality of the management of patients with COVID-19. The overwhelming access to namely evidence-based information had the limitation of insufficient time to screen from among all sources those papers that met the scientific rigor process to validate the results. The above and the rapidly changing information on the physiopathology and the treatment of COVID-19, had a negative effect on the trust from implementers of the guidelines. The health system is faced with changes in guidelines from the traditional 3–5 years to changes every week, every month.

Risk communication plan

A fundamental objective of risk communication is to reduce and contain harm in a crisis. In the case of a pandemic, risk communication plan is the best way to prevent, contain, and mitigate the spread of contagion. Within the process of developing a risk communication plan, a pivotal aspect remains the definition of areas of communication for the different beneficiaries. For this, the team conducting this process has to be knowledgeable of the target population to determine the clear, precise, and concise messages to aid in the development of new behaviors to stop the spread of the disease. In risk communication, there is no one-size-fits-all. While the expected outcome is universal, the how varies by population groups.

Conclusion

The fight against the global COVID-19 pandemic cannot be left to the health system. The fight needs to be carried out in all settings outside of the health system. A country can effectively contain the transmission of the virus from human to human if every individual is compliant with transmission precaution measures known to be effective. It is not a government's only responsibility, it's an individual responsibility vis-a-vis the human being wired to be interconnected with other individuals.

Lockdown as a public health measure

12

Laila Woc-Colburn[a] and Daniel Godinez[b]

[a]Division of Infectious Diseases, Emory University School of Medicine, Atlanta, GA, United States,
[b]Internal Medicine, Belize Healthcare Partners Limited, Belize City, Belize

As we learned through this book, coronavirus disease 2019 (COVID-19) pandemic brought to light how vulnerable we are to the infectious respiratory virus due to our living patterns, travel, and housing. To curb down the spread of severe acute respiratory syndrome coronavirus 2 (SARS-CoV-2), the implementation of public health mitigation strategies was necessary. One of them was the lockdowns and quarantine policies throughout the world. What is a quarantine vs lockdown? How effective are they? How long and how often do we need them? Do they have an impact on our overall health? These are some of the questions that we will explore in this chapter.

The most basic public health tool is to quarantine, followed by the lockdown. Quarantine as defined by Webster dictionary as "a state, period, or place of isolation in which people or animals that have arrived from elsewhere or been exposed to the infectious or contagious disease are placed"[1] and lockdown as "a temporary condition imposed by governmental authorities (as during the outbreak of an epidemic disease) in which people are required to stay in their homes and refrain from or limit activities outside the home involving public contact (such as dining out or attending large gatherings)."[2]

These are public health measures design to slow down the spread of infections. We have used these tools throughout history and implemented them during epidemics dating back to the Plague of Justinian (527–565 CE).[3] Boccaccio wrote the most famous quarantine/lockdown, The Decameron. The Decameron is a compilation of stories told by Florentines escaping the plague to pass the Renaissance. Quarantines have been implemented since then overtime when an infectious disease poses a threat. In our recent past, the most memorable quarantine has been Ebola in 2014, H1N1 in 2009, and SARS in 2003. We have not experienced the magnitude of this pandemic since 1917 with influenza.

The concept of starting a lockdown was first implemented in Wuhan, China, in January 2020 by the Chinese Centers for Disease Control and Prevention to prevent its spread throughout China. At that time, SARS-CoV-2 had high infectivity of 2.5 people per case (reproductive number R_0) and a case fatality rate of 4.4%. Due to its high transmissibility as a respiratory virus, the idea of lockdown was to help stop and slow down its spread. This measure was quickly adopted by most of the world against

COVID-19 Pandemic. https://doi.org/10.1016/B978-0-323-82860-4.00013-6

the spread of SARS-CoV-2 from Asia to Europe to the Americas. Some of the lockdown measures implemented by governments included[4]:

- curfews
- gathering restrictions (limiting the size or canceling them)
- isolation at home (including attending work, school, etc.)
- restriction of movement of their citizen to the only essentials
- travel restrictions

Although the lockdown has its advantages in decreasing new cases, mortality is not without its challenges.

Advantages

The significant advantage of the lockdown, when there are no vaccines or treatments, is slowing down the disease in the naïve population and decreasing its mortality. It gives the city or country officials' time to develop strategies that will help contain the disease, especially if there are no health-care infrastructures or capacity to perform testing for surveillance.[5] Other indirect advantages of the global lockdown were decreasing pollution levels, increasing flora and fauna, telecommuting, and telehealth.

As the lockdown phase shows decreasing rates or plateauing of the cases, this is the time to reconsider the reopening or unlocking stage. Due to the incubation period of SARS-CoV-2, 14–21 days can be used to start reopening strategies. Examples of countries with successful reopening are New Zealand, South Korea, and Taiwan.[6] The reopening should continue mitigation practices, including social distancing, face mask wearing, digital contract tracing, serosurveillance studies, and vaccination.[6]

Challenges

Despite deaccelerating the COVID-19 pandemic, the lockdowns themselves had various adverse effects on health (physical and mental), education, social interaction, economic productivity, and nutrition. Lockdowns are not meant to be a long-term solution but short term and serve as bridges to contact tracing, treatment, and vaccination. In the last year, the lockdown was used to control the number of cases and in some countries lasted for several weeks or went into a second or third lockdown. Here are some of the significant challenges faced by the 2020 COVID-19 lockdown.

Economic effects

Since the start of the COVID-19 pandemic, the world went into recession and is facing a global crisis. As the world went into lockdown and the demand for personal protective equipment was on the rise, supply shortages occurred from increasing prices to food shortages at the grocery stores.

The disruption to the flights and factories in mainland China had a harmful effect due to delays in manufacturing electronic equipment, pharmaceuticals, and food. The stock market fell in the early months of the pandemic but recover with the news of possible treatment and vaccines. The impact on the travel and leisure industry was unimaginable. The world of travel was double impacted by the reduction of flights and the cancellations of cruises. It is estimated that more than 60% of restaurants won't be able to reopen. Just as the restaurant business went down, so did retail business at the shopping centers due to the lockdown restrictions. Unemployment rose, which lead to increase sexual exploitation, homelessness, and food insecurity.

Mental and psychological effects

The lockdown measures did globally disrupt the daily lives of all the people living in the world. The daily tasks and mundane routines ceased to exist and were replaced by restrictions and monotony, sometimes. The change in pattern and isolation lead to people feeling more anxious and less in control of their lives. The isolation leads to an increased number of psychological disorders like acute stress disorders, irritability, insomnia, emotional distress and mood disorders, depression, fear and panic, anxiety and stress because of financial concerns, frustration, boredom, loneliness, lack of supplies, and poor communication.[4] People already have mental illness were more vulnerable. Food insufficiency had increased during the COVID-19 pandemic and affected vulnerable populations, placing individuals at higher risk for poor mental health symptoms.

A study was done by Serafini et al.[7] showed that the most relevant psychological reactions to COVID-19 infection were uncontrolled fears related to illness, pervasive anxiety, frustration, and boredom, disabling loneliness. More resilient people had better coping mechanisms, and good social support had fewer psychological effects. Strong support networks and coping mechanisms help lessen anxiety and depression.

Social inequities

COVID-19 brought to light the social inequities that exist today in the world. The social and economic determinants of health were influenced by low income, access to health care, and access to food.[8]

In the United States of America, the African-American and Latino communities were impacted the most by COVID-19.

The social inequities were due to lack of health care, preexisting conditions, essential jobs (not medical), and structural inequality.

Future

COVID-19 pandemic is an unprecedented event in our lifetime, where we had to take draconian measures to stop the spread of the virus. Where lockdowns a good mitigation measure? Countries like New Zealand, South Korea, and Taiwan would agree since they use the time to strengthen their health-care systems, continue with public health measures such as masking, social distancing, and contact tracing. In summary, the continued use of epidemiological surveillance to appropriately calibrate social distancing efforts and to achieve a low and stable infection rate, thereby minimizing overall morbidity and mortality, is a reliable long-term approach to follow and maintain until the COVID-19 pandemic reaches its herd immunity with vaccination.

References

1. quarantine. In: *Merriam-Webster.com*. Merriam-Webster; 2021. Web. 18 Feb 2021.
2. lockdown. In: *Merriam-Webster.com*. Merriam-Webster; 2021. Web. 18 Feb 2021.
3. Bassareo PP, Melis MR, Marras S, et al. Learning from the past in the COVID-19 era: rediscovery of quarantine, previous pandemics, origin of hospitals and national healthcare systems, and ethics in medicine. *Postgrad Med J*. 2020;96:633–638.
4. Usher K, Bhullar N, Jackson D. Life in the pandemic: social isolation and mental health. *J Clin Nurs*. 2020;29:2756–2757. https:/doi.org/10.1111/jocn.15290.
5. Lytras T, Tsiodras S. Lockdowns and the COVID-19 pandemic: what is the endgame? *Scand J Public Health*. 2021;49(1):37–40. https:/doi.org/10.1177/1403494820961293.
6. Jung F, Krieger V, Hufert FT, Küpper JH. How we should respond to the Coronavirus SARS-CoV-2 outbreak: A German perspective. *Clin Hemorheol Microcirc*. 2020;74(4): 363–372. https:/doi.org/10.3233/CH-209004.
7. Serafini G, Parmigiani B, Amerio A, Aguglia A, Sher L, Amore M. The psychological impact of COVID-19 on the mental health in the general population. *QJM*. 2020; 113:531–537.
8. Clark E, Fredricks K, Woc-Colburn L, Bottazzi ME, Weatherhead J. Disproportionate impact of the COVID-19 pandemic on immigrant communities in the United States. *PLoS Negl Trop Dis*. 2020;14(7):e0008484. https:/doi.org/10.1371/journal.pntd.0008484.

Politics and the pandemic 13

Michael Singh

Office of the Prime Minister of Belize, Belmopan, Belize

In this Information Age, the value of science as the leading source for public policy on health has largely been replaced with the mood of the masses, and from the need of political leaders to respond, partly to save their political fortunes. With the majority of governments, the goal of reducing the spread of diseases like the coronavirus and keeping people safe has taken a back seat to politics.

This delicate balance plays itself out on a daily basis, and in an instant, with new outlets blaring a loud and obnoxious combination of opinions and facts, often directed in an effort to tip opinion in favor of their favorite political cause. With major elections looming on the horizon in the United States and other countries, the politicization of the pandemic has become a convenient narrative by candidates, their support base, and the media, with the aim to credit or discredit the efforts of political leaders in implementing a domestically homogeneous respond, much less one—a global one.

In this modern political landscape, several factors have and will continue to impact the global outcome: the fatality rates and the economic fallout and recovery from the pandemic. I wish to highlight four of the main factors and will describe them, their impact, and an outlook as to how these factors will change as the pandemic progresses. These four factors, such as globalization, technology, ideology, and inequality, are intricately intertwined and in fact form the basis for the pervasive political movements that impact the policy responses that unfold before our eyes on a daily basis.

Some 2000 years ago, true globalization began as luxury goods from China started to find their way to Rome, once the capital of the Western world, via the Silk Road. Coincidentally, much of the Roman empire was undergoing a metamorphosis that culminated in the move toward its fragmentation and its eventual conversion into the Holy Roman Empire, eventually leading to the rooting of the philosophy of Christianity in Western daily life, which has, since that era, formed the basis of many political movements. This global spreading of goods, people, services, and philosophy that flourished over the last 2000 years has perhaps faced its greatest challenge and, at the same time, found its most powerful fuel over the last century, as advances in discovery, technology, and information has propelled science to the forefront of human consciousness, effectively upending the traditional dominance of religious ideology.

COVID-19 Pandemic. https://doi.org/10.1016/B978-0-323-82860-4.00011-2

I say, this amazing phenomenon of accelerated change has caused us as humans to question every facet of our lives upon which our faith and our fortunes have been based.

The year 2020 has become symbolic of a perfect political storm. A storm where in the midst of a pandemic, the most fundamental clash of culture and counterculture, liberal vs conservative, and North vs South is occurring. This global resurgence in civil rights, this cry for racial equality, and this challenge of traditional law enforcement could not have come at a more pivotal time and at a time when governments are struggling with pandemic response and the economic fallout caused by the unprecedented phenomenon of a crash in global supply and demand.

Like every other factor in human development, globalization has also accelerated with the advancement in science, technology, and information over the past 100 years. With it has come an explosion in human interaction through travel and through electronic exchanges of ideas and transactions. Language barriers and distance have been canceled out by a connected global education system and by improved and lower-cost transportation. This shrinking of our world has brought humans closer together physically and figuratively, creating the perfect conduit upon which new and deadly viruses like the coronavirus have conveniently hitched a ride for its great world tour.

This novel hitchhiker was predicted, but the complications of our modern world were never factored into the equation. It is important to point out that for the 5 years prior to 2020, there has been a global move toward nationalism, which has seen a new breed of world leaders take the centre stage in the world's largest economies. Leaders like Donald Trump in the United States, Jair Bolsonaro in Brazil, and Andrés Manual López Obrador in Mexico have taken extreme nationalistic stances to push a new brand of populism in a democratic context. The mass movements fuelled by the resulting polarization of citizens in these countries have become a fertile ground for the use of and conversely the manipulation of facts and science with an aim to appeal to the extreme bases.

In the United States, the left leaning media has hyped the pandemic, and their analysis of the response by the White House has become a very powerful vehicle to discredit the Trump administration. For their part, the Trump campaign has itself subtly encouraged a rejection of scientific-based advice on coronavirus disease 2019 (COVID-19), including the outright rejection of mask wearing, along with a campaign to prematurely reopen states and cities, despite scientific and health advice to the contrary. This polarization of diverse groups by both sides of the political landscape, and the politicization of the pandemic has seriously thwarted the efforts of the health managers to present a unified message to the general public. Even more seriously, the mixed message from the White House, and the refusal of the administration to provide federal directives, and instead to cede authority and final decisions on COVID-19 policy to the state governors, has led to uneven responses.

The holy grail of any pandemic response is to flatten the curve. That is, employing coordinated efforts by the government and the public to reduce the infection rate in order that medical systems, research, and readiness can get ahead of the inevitable rush that comes from a large number of ill persons.[1] In a situation where mixed signals are given by those that govern and where political polarization among citizens is prevalent, the ability to achieve the flattening of the curve becomes ever more difficult. In the case of these countries, the populist messages and the very example of the actions of popular leaders have caused an immediate spike in the curve after quarantine efforts have been eased.

The lack of coordination on COVID-19 response policy inside nations has led to an even more difficult situation in a globalized world. While much of Europe, Canada, and Asia and countless smaller dependent nations have been successful in flattening their curve, the fact that large trading and tourism source markets like the United States and Brazil has led to severe travel restrictions against citizens of those countries. The United States, traditionally a gold mine of high spending tourists, has effectively become a virtual leper colony, with a pervasive fear in destination management that they are inviting the importation of new infections.

From the early days of the pandemic, travel and leisure has fallen to a level where airlines, cruise lines, hotels, and restaurants can no longer cover their operating costs much less make a profit. This temporary shutdown was to have ended with a coordinated and managed reopening, whereby companies bolstered by government aid can restart services with a move toward full operation under new management guidelines. International passenger carriers have thrived with globalization from open movements of mass numbers of passengers across states and international borders. The halting of these movements by much of the world has left an unprecedented number of airplanes and cruise ships idle, stripping billions from the valuations of these companies, and massive layoffs of employees. In acts of desperation, global carriers have chosen to push the envelope and to announce a continuation of travel services, despite the severe drop in demand resulting from increasing cost of compliance and screening, traveler fear, and personal economic uncertainties.

The standard protocol of pandemic control of a respiratory disease requires the controlling of distances among people in order to slow infection spreads while waiting for science and medical responses to catch up with vaccines and hospital capacity. This temporary environment is in direct conflict with a world that was built on maximizing the carrying capacity of humans in aircraft, cruise ships, concerts, public transports, offices, and residential structures. As the norm of maximum capacity gets interrupted, so do the profits from it, and when profits get interrupted in a capitalist society, politicians are compelled to act, often in desperation, as the need for earning slowly starts to override the ideal for public health and wellness.

Globally interconnected market forces and financial markets react to the changes in demand and the damage to profitability, as we see the incomes of major industries evaporate before our very eyes. Entertainment, sports, travel, and leisure have been on virtual shutdowns with hundreds of millions of employees worldwide out of work. Predictions by economists of doom have prompted political leaders to weigh the risks of mortality of a relatively small percentage of the global population against the long-term damage from economic recession. This conflict plays itself out on every news outlet, where messages from science-based pandemic managers like the Centers for

Disease Control in the United States, conflict with the messages from the White House on a daily basis. In the United States, this confusion has had a marked impact on the growth in new cases and in mortality rates, making that country the new epicenter for COVID-19.

In Brazil, the approach by President Jairo Bolsonaro has been even more radical, and the statistics have shown similar results to the United States. Early presidential rhetoric that contradicted science, along with images of the President void of personal protection, while openly criticizing their use, have led to an uneven adoption of best practices by the general population. Likewise, in Mexico, the government continued business as usual, not opting for lockdowns or border closures, and as of today, Mexico is considered to have the fastest growth in cases in the world.

Perhaps the worst outcome of the political challenges to controlling the pandemic has been the sharp divide among political supporters in those polarized nations. In the United States, the wearing of masks has become a statement of political preference instead of a health measure, and the packing of stadiums for political rallies with barefaced throngs of shouting supporters fly in the face of proper quarantine protocols.

The impact of technology in today's world has been perhaps the greatest catalyst of change, and perhaps the most important defining factor compared to pandemics from past centuries. The forefront of this has been the great advances in information technology. The movement of news and updates from across the world occurs in seconds, and the person to person sharing of information in an instant at all levels of society and by all demographics has kept the world informed and forewarned. This has also, to some extent, led to significant movement of misinformation, hype, and the spread of ideology that has hampered the response to COVID-19.

The movement of information about virus spreads from its beginnings in Wuhan, China, was a lot faster than the movement of the actual virus, which gave health authorities the ability to prepare and to react more effectively.

Information movement, however, is only the tip of the technological advances that have helped governments to respond to the COVID-19 pandemic threat. As the disease travels around the world and as infections and deaths increase, many governments are turning to technology to help to flatten the curve. Some fear, however, that the use of technology, in particular those aimed at tracking or controlling citizens, may be a harbinger of a Big Brother future that has been well portrayed by Hollywood over the years. This dilemma between health response and freedom is yet another battle that is being waged and a situation that preoccupies political leaders in this pandemic era.

Several countries including Singapore, South Korea, Taiwan, and even Germany and Israel are using the global positioning system (GPS) via mobile phones to track the movements of people and to enforce quarantines against the natural urge of people to move freely. South Korea has gone so far as to combine GPS tracking with credit card activity and surveillance footage to trace the movements of persons who may be infected or may be in contact with the virus. Some countries have adopted a mandatory use of a tracking wristband for arriving visitors as a means to enforcing quarantine rules and to track their movements when in country. Even more extreme measures are being employed with the use of drones for surveillance, to disinfect public areas, to remotely monitor body temperatures, and to police the movements of people within managed corridors.

The thought of this new electronically controlled police state is a frightening one, if one were to remove the pandemic from the equation. The use of artificial intelligence for instance to capture and analyze data and to provide recommendations to policy makers on actions invokes images from the dystopian future portrayed in the movie, the Matrix, and provides a ripe ground for conspiracy theorists and libertarians to raise alarms. In a pandemic, however, justification for the technology is more easily achieved, and these advances are therefore slowly finding their way into society, approved by political leaders, as tools to combat the virus and to help society to return to normal. This choice between Big Brother surveillance and an uncontrolled spread of the virus has become perhaps one of the greatest one for society to make in this modern era, as the aftermath of this technology use may in fact have a more profound impact on our future than the pandemic itself.

So, what happens after the health crisis is over? As with any technological shift, people will eventually become comfortable with its existence and presence in our daily lives. The traditional practice of confidentiality in managing health data suddenly becomes blurred as personal and public health data converges in the need for case management, to conduct contact tracing, and to isolate and quarantine individuals who are deemed as risky to the community. The more people contract the disease, the less will be the stigma placed on those with the infection, and the less important will be the need to keep that information confidential.

The need for social isolation will also encourage the growth of telemedicine technology. Remote monitoring will expand to include smart devices connected to remote monitoring technology that will allow patients to be "seen" by a doctor who is not present. The ability to monitor vital signs and even administer medication will become a norm, again raising questions of data security, cyber invasions, and personal privacy.

Even more innocuous forms of technology are being propelled due to the COVID-19 threat. In developing countries, governments are scrambling to accelerate the development of digital services not only to minimize physical interactions but also to bring more efficiency to government. This movement toward digitization is being followed by private enterprises that find the need to deliver goods and services to a home-bound population. The proliferation of online vendors, new payment, and delivery systems using technology is spawning a boom in the sale of technology and in innovation, and perhaps for the first time in the world's history, the infrastructure for technological connectivity is as important as the physical infrastructure of a nation.

This rapid transformation of nations into the digital realm also brings major challenges for political leaders in developing countries. Legislation has to be updated in many respects as most governments services are designed on paper-based analog systems, and direct online citizen access requires new technologies like cloud computing, internet protocols, and strong encryption. Beyond this, the concept of digital signatures can only work if national identification and authentications frameworks are strong, and online transactions only work with trustworthy and efficient electronic payments systems. Even in the United States, the deployment of the unemployment benefits to the burgeoning ranks of displaced workers due to the pandemic has been less than ideal, with workers standing in long lines in defiance to quarantine orders to register for and inquire about their benefits. In other countries where financial inclusion is low, the registration for and distribution of aid and food packages became a monumental task.

Technology for the management of the actual pandemic has also seen a surge. The ability to manage the mass amounts of data gathered from contact tracing activities and to use that data effectively is a task that is difficult for human teams. For this reason, the development of data systems to gather, disseminate, utilize, and analyze health data to inform political decisions has become a key in this fight against the virus. Due to fundamental rights governing privacy, most nations with highly developed democracies have been slow to adopt technologies to support the invasive efforts needed for contact tracing.

Even the efforts from Google and Apple have been measured with a great deal of caution and awareness of privacy. These tech giants teamed up and entered the equation by developing apps on their platform that would allow individuals to conduct proximity tracking and tracing. That is to say, to allow individual to monitor their surroundings for the presence of infected persons in order to avoid making contact or to make a decision to self-isolate. Their efforts have clashed with governments like the United Kingdom who initially rejected the use of these technologies in their contact tracing efforts because those companies would not provide data to government health managers but eventually reverted to the Google/Apple platform after spending millions on their own solution that could not pass the test for privacy and security.

The pandemic has caused people to turn to technology more and more to manage their daily lives for staying connected with family and friends, for working remotely, to learn, to access medical care, and even as a conduit to deliver food and other necessary supplies. This potential to bring us closer together and to make us safer, healthier, and happier, as promised by the architects of this Information Age, is being realized in a rapid manner in front of our eyes. On the other hand, never before have we been as challenged to ensure reliability in that connectivity, as it is no longer a novelty, but a necessity. The risk of attacks on our privacy as a result of increased surveillance by governments and the potential misuse of data for malice or for profit are more prevalent today, yet we must learn how to balance those risks against the benefits to be gained in this and future fights against viruses that can cause pandemics.

Political leaders are on the front line in charting the safe path for the use of technology in this pandemic era. It means that they must take steps to ensure universal access to technology by all, from every child who's only choice for education is online to the infirm that needs access to virtual health care in a physical system that is overburdened due to COVID-19 spikes. The balance between ethics, inequality, and policy overreach as we adopt this new way of living is perhaps one of the most important debate that has to be had as we maneuver this challenge.[2]

It is apparent that conservative political ideology may have delayed protective policy implementation and promoted the spread of COVID-19 in the United States.[3] Similar outcomes have been revealed in Brazil, Mexico, and in some countries in Europe, where political ideology has polarized citizens and political lines are drawn between liberal and conservative political camps.

The politicization of COVID-19 in the United States has played a key role in the virus's proliferation, with conservatives feeling less concerned about the virus than liberals as a result of President Donald Trump's downplaying the pandemic's urgency.[4] On the other side, the anti-Trump media has not lost a moment in highlighting the president's failures and missteps in relation to the pandemic, often ridiculing his gaffes and actions, personifying him as the face of pandemic failure. While his approach encouraged anti-quarantine sentiment and behavior among his followers, the media onslaught served as reinforcement for them to be even more stubborn against quarantine measures and to latch on to baseless conspiracy theories to bolster their arguments.

The problem with this political drama is that the fact that lives are at risk seems to be a backdrop to a presidential campaign, on one side to reinforce ideology and on the other hand to depose possibly one of the most polarizing figures in American political history.

Along with this polarized view of COVID-19 in free democracies, there is a marked rise in belief in conspiracy theories about the disease and the pandemic in general, widely shared via social media platforms.

A study by King's College published in the Journal of Psychological Medicine finds that people who get their news from social media sources are more likely to break lockdown rules.[5] The researchers tested seven statements about COVID-19, revealing the following levels of belief:

- Three in 10 (30%) think coronavirus was probably created in a laboratory, up from a quarter (25%) at the beginning of April.
- Three in 10 (28%) think most people in the United Kingdom have already had coronavirus without realizing it.
- Three in 10 (30%) believe the COVID-19 death toll is being deliberately reduced or hidden by the authorities.
- One in seven (14%) believe the death toll is being deliberately exaggerated by the authorities.
- One in eight (13%) believe that the current pandemic is part of a global effort to force everyone to be vaccinated.
- More than one in 20 (8%) believe that the symptoms that most people blame on COVID-19 appear to be connected to 5G network radiation.
- More than one in 20 (7%) believe there is no hard evidence that COVID-19 really exists.

In his analysis of the study, Professor Bobby Duffy wrote, "there are clear links between belief in conspiracies and both lower trust in government and less compliance with the guidelines set to control the disease. Where people get their information about the virus is also strongly related, with both believing in conspiracies and breaking the lockdown rules clearly linked to getting more of your information from social media."[6]

In such an environment, it becomes extremely difficult for political leaders who are seeking reelection to stick hard and fast to facts and science in their rhetoric. The ability to educate such a large swath of the population in sufficient time in order that the rules for quarantine and pandemic management can be properly enforced becomes extremely difficult. In China and other Asian nations that are accustomed to authoritarian imposed public health, the compliance has been much higher.

In the United States, the front line of this ideological war sits with the policy of wearing masks. While it is widely accepted that this practice contributed greatly to the flattening of the curve in the 1918 Spanish flu pandemic, adverse ideology has equated mask wearing with political preference, with curtailing of freedoms, and in general with being a liberal vs a conservative. This growing pandemic of ideology, and the fact that the United States is now the epicenter of the global pandemic with no signs that their second curve will slow down, is a major concern in the rest of the world, particularly in the Western Hemisphere. In this hemisphere, infections are spreading rapidly through Latin America and the Caribbean into South America, effectively devastating the already fragile economies of the region.

The actual direct impact of COVID-19 is only now just being felt, with every country in the world feeling either the impacts on their health systems or on their economy. At some point when the pandemic eases, the entire human family will have to live with its effects for years to come, but the costs will not be the same for all. While COVID-19 has respected no border, even after its gone, it will continue to discriminate against the most vulnerable.

The predictions are alarming. The United Nations Development Program (UNDP) expects that for the first time since prior to 1990, the global human development index, a combined measure of the world's education, health, and living conditions, will decline this year. This decline will occur in every region. Global per capita income is expected to fall by 4%, and the World Bank has warned that the impact of the virus could push between 40 and 60 million people into extreme poverty this year, with sub-Saharan Africa and South Asia being the hardest hit.[7]

The International Labour Organization estimates that half of working people could lose their jobs in just 6 months of the crisis, and the virus could cost the global economy about US$10 trillion this year alone.[8]

COVID-19 is exposing the gap between the haves and the have-nots. In the developed world, the wealthy have had the luxury of quarantining in their vacation homes and on private yachts, while poor displaced workers with school children risk being evicted from cramped rental apartments. The payment of economic relief has also been slow in coming, and the spread of the relief itself is discriminatory, with little going to small businesses, resulting in mass business failures due to the prolonged shutdown.

Inequality, however, is on the most prominent display as we look at the ability of nations to respond to the crisis. Early on, in the scramble for scarce medical supplies, diversion of equipment and supplies destined for small vulnerable nations by the United States became a policy, even resulting in seizures during transit. In poor over-populated nations like India and other parts of Asia, millions of displaced workers were forced to walk for days to return to their home villages, with many sleeping in the open with unsanitary conditions because there are no resources to assist them.

The disparity in medical capacity has also come into sharp focus. According to UNDP data, the most developed countries have 55 hospital beds, more than 30 doctors, and 81 nurses for every 10,000 people. By contrast, in the less developed countries, there are only 7 beds, 2.5 doctors, and 6 nurses for the same number of people. And as previously pointed out, lockdowns have made the digital divide more obvious, with billions of people who have no access to electricity or running water, much less the internet, which shuts them out from being able to interact with family or to participate in the new norm of online learning.

With schools' closure and the divides in distance learning, UNDP estimates indicate that 86% of primary school-age children in low human development countries are currently not getting an education, compared to just 20% in countries with very high human development.

With schools closed, UNDP estimates that effective out of school rates could regress to levels not seen since the 1980s—the largest reversal ever—taking us back to a time before the Sustainable Development Goals or even the Millennium Development Goals and threatening the hard work and progress of the past 30 years.

The great economic pandemic is the looming challenge that all nations will face, but none more profoundly than developing nations. For governments, this challenge will be further exacerbated by the fragility of their economies and the debt levels that they have had to manage even before the pandemic.

The international monetary fund (IMF) estimates that the cost of the global response so far includes fiscal actions amounting to almost $11 trillion to contain the pandemic and its damage to the economy as well as central bank actions amounting to over $6 trillion. The share of this burden in developed countries is enormous; however, those countries' ability to borrow these massive numbers comes simply from their capacity to increase their money supply with hardly any impact on their creditworthiness. In the case of developing countries, however, the capacity to borrow is severely constrained by ratios that only apply in their case, with an ever-looming threat that falling currency values and international credit ratings will signal instant Armageddon.

In this reality where productivity is down, and where both demand and supply are on the ropes at the same time, government policy has to be carefully assessed. Debt ceilings that propelled growth 5 years ago are no longer valid, and risk assessment cannot be done using the same metrics. Until institutions like the IMF and others make these adjustments, however, the developing world must rely principally on dwindling credit and on the charity of friendly nations in order that they can meet the demands for basic health, food, and shelter by its residents.

Those nations that are reliant on tourism, like most of the smaller Caribbean nations, face the greatest risk. Not only are they vulnerable from imported COVID-19 infections in the short term, but also the disappearance of overnight and cruise tourism poses an even greater risk of economic regression, mass unemployment, and social unrest.

In the COVID-19 era, our present preoccupation with the management of the pandemic is only the beginning of the challenges facing governments across the globe. This era will require a new version of political will. Never before has political leadership been challenged as it will be in the next few years.

References

1. Chris Kenyon, Flattening-the-Curve associated with reduced COVID-19 case fatality rates—an ecological analysis of 65 countries, n.d.
2. Morris S. *Technology Can Play a Role in Managing COVID-19, but we must get the policies right.* www.newamerica.org.
3. D. Rosenfield. Political Ideology and the Outbreak of COVID-19 in the United States, n.d.
4. Kushner Gadarian S, Goodman SW, Pepinsky TB. *Partisanship, Health Behavior and the Policy Attitudes in the Early Stages of the COVID-19 Pandemic*; 2020.
5. Allington D, Duffy B, Wessely S, Dhavan N, Rubin J. Health-protective behaviour, social media usage and conspiracy belief during the COVID-19 public health emergency. *Psychol Med.* 2020;1–7. https://doi.org/10.1017/S003329172000224X.
6. Professor Bobby Duffy, Director of the Policy Institute at King's College London, n.d.
7. UNDP. Coronavirus vs. inequality, May 2020. https://feature.undp.org/coronavirus-vs-inequality/.
8. ILO. International Labour Organization (ILO) Monitor. COVID-19 and the World of Work. ed.; 2021 (Updated estimates and analysis). 7th ed.

The effects of the pandemic on oil services and shipping industry

14

William G. MacDonald

The British East India Company Limited, Birkenhead, Merseyside, United Kingdom

Introduction

Oil and gas industry have experienced *déjà vu* as oil prices have once again crashed, this time due to the destruction of demand associated with coronavirus disease 2019 (COVID-19) and the war on prices between Russia and Saudi Arabia and other Organization of the Petroleum Exporting Countries members.

What path lies ahead for the industry in the coming months and years? This chapter discovers some of the facts that exist around the trading of oil products, their transport, and the value set at the international markets. We air some thoughts (and some questions) to help oil and gas companies navigate the current landscape.

Surprisingly, it seems there is still very little publicity or knowledge of the highly technical operations of modern ships, as well as the crew who sail them.

There are over 50,000 ships plying the oceans of the world at any one given time. About 1 million highly trained seamen are employed at sea, while a further 1 million take their home leave.

Generally, seamen are required to commit to work aboard their ship for long periods at a time, seldom less than 6 months. They disembark in some parts of the world, travel home, have a leave period of 6–8 weeks and then rejoin another ship in another part of the world.

The first known records of sea vessels chronicle their use of oars and sail. The first sea-going sailing ships were developed by the Austronesian people in what is now called Southern China and Taiwan. They invented catamarans and outriggers. Their claw sails made it conceivable for them to begin making long voyages into open ocean origination what it was the foundation of the Austronesian Expansion at around 3000–1500 BCE.

From those remote times to the actual moment, sailing in general and the transport of merchandise in ships has certainly evolved. The advances in all aspects of shipping have continued. Modern technology has, for example, completely revolutionized marine communications and navigation. The Internet has radically changed how shipping companies trade with their clients. Although the ships of today bear little resemblance to those originally developed, they continue to share the same

COVID-19 Pandemic. https://doi.org/10.1016/B978-0-323-82860-4.00019-7

purpose of transporting goods throughout the world from one place to another while being manned by a skilled mariners who leave behind their homes and families.

Experts advise us that more than 90% of goods worldwide are transported by ships. Shipping, then, is the main transporting method of goods and the vertebral column of the world trade. Without it, the present-day economy could not be sustained.

The oil industry and shipping

Crude and clean refined oil (gasoline, diesel, kerosene, and gas oil) are carried on board oil tankers to and from oil production platforms, oil terminals, and oil refineries. They are delivered to tankage in all parts of the world. The slots allocated for any ship at port are limited and continuously subject to demand and rapid turnover. In a similar fashion to a busy airport, trading ports in the world, as well as those near refineries or oil industry, are given timely and many times require several days of waiting time offshore prior to allowing docking time. Because time spent in port to deliver to tankage is very short, seldom more than 36 hours, and given other procedures such as compulsory and very necessary inspections by officials also take place in port, it is an extremely busy time for everyone to ensure the ship is loaded or discharged as quickly as possible in order to meet time limitations; consequently, there is very rarely an opportunity for any crew member to ever go ashore for even a short period.

Captains and ships officers are permanently under pressure to save time and reduce costs. It is said that "*a ship in port Burns money, a ship at sea Earns money*"

Thus the urgent necessity for achieving a fast turnaround in ports and oil terminals is constantly the call of the day.

The effects of COVID-19 on oil services, oil logistics, and shipping industries

As the spread of the COVID-19 progressed from China to other countries, the problems for our industry, as it happened to others, increased. We were fighting on two fronts dealing with an oil price war and a pandemic. The dropping price in oil was dramatic. On January 1, a barrel of crude oil sold for $67.05 on New York's NASDAQ exchange. In early March, it was trading at around $30.00 per barrel.

Any reserve stored on tanks of oil companies became worth, approximately a half of what they had previously been worth at the start of the year. As companies struggled with this cut in their values, the situation became worse as the entire sector was overwhelmed by the huge downfall in the demand, the closedown of the aviation sector (one of the prime consumers of refined oil worldwide), industrial slowdowns, travel restrictions, stricter immigration regulations, requirements for quarantine, and border closures with major restrictions to worldwide trade.

Understandably, agents were reluctant to travel to oil terminals. The authorities began finding it increasingly difficult to man or safely provide the services required to berth large supertankers. Supplies of food and water and any provision to the tankers were also compromised.

Travel restrictions meant that seamen could not travel to join ships, thus those aboard who had finished their contracted period were not only unable to be relieved or leave the ship, there were no flights available for them to travel home to their families. By May 2020, it was estimated that 150,000 seamen were stranded aboard their vessels, not allowed to leave the ship at all.

Merchant vessels do not carry a doctor, there are no hospitals in the Atlantic, Pacific, or Indian Oceans. This form of confinement, combined with the fear of contracting COVID-19, can of course be hazardous to the mental health of the crew members. At any time on a ship, captains and ship officers have the duty to care for their crew and for their morale, and teamwork is of utmost importance. Working in a close space for a long period of time in many times hostile weather conditions and perilous environments can be a hazard by itself. This becomes even more challenging when considering the fear associated to the pandemic, the limitations for the seamen to return home, or even to leave the ship ashore. Although these highly trained individuals are experts in their profession, they are not doctors. Throughout this period, a great deal of added pressure has been put upon them.

Economic impact of the lockdown on oil services, oil logistics, and shipping industry

Demand for oil plunged as COVID-19 caused people to lockdown in their homes, stop driving, or traveling any distance to and from work. Transport in general was radically reduced. Airlines closed. We saw the lowest oil prices in almost two decades, with worse predicted to come or at least to be prolonged throughout significant time.

The dramatic drop in oil price negatively affected the returns on exploration projects and caused many future proposed explorations to be cancelled.

Tanker rates, instead of dropping, as initially predicted, rose, especially for large tankers; this was because the oil majors wanted to fill all of their tanks and storage them in places with cheaply priced oil. As soon as prices decreased, oil companies sailed their tankers to be filled with cheaply priced oil and anchored them in safe areas approximately 50 miles offshore. By mid-May 2020, there were about 40 large tankers anchored offshore California, with an equal number in the North Sea, West Africa, the Far East, and the Arabian Gulf.

The effect of the oil glut on the world

Most laymen innocently welcome cheap oil and cheap energy. However, this cheap energy comes with its own problems.

The year 2019 was the first year in which the USA exported crude oil. Small crude oil producers were busily pumping oil from small oil wells in Texas,

Oklahoma, and other states, also fracking for crude oil became big business. Break-even costs for fracking are very much higher than the costs of cheap crude oil from the Middle East. Consequently, those small oil producers were eventually put out of business, oil exports from the USA slowed down or stopped and cheap imported oil became popular.

Small oil-producing countries such as Ecuador, Columbia, and Trinidad, whose only real means of earning hard currency is by exporting crude oil, are now really suffering as they struggle to service their debt. Many of their workforce have lost their jobs with consequent impact on their economy.

The future

As the pandemic continues abating the world and no solution is seen in the near future, the situation for the oil industry will likely continue, and this will translate into Tanker Rates remaining high until the end of the year 2020. Then, if, hopefully, the COVID-19 virus slows down enough to enable the world to, progressively, begin to get back to where we were before, we might be able to return to the previously present scenario.

After summer (2020), I expect the freight rates to drop back down again because the oil inventories are being used up, and oil prices will then start to climb up again.

As to COVID-19, I leave that opinion to the good doctors and scientists who are desperately trying to find a vaccine. Personally, I believe that COVID-19 will be with us for a long time, and that eventually, humans will develop a natural immunity to this virus. The world, although changed, will continue as it has done for billions of years, and ships and shipping will continue, as before, carrying the vast majority of all the worlds commodities, from one country to another, as it is the safest and most cost-effective means of transport.

Disclaimer

The views expressed are solely of the author, and ETEnergyworld.com does not necessarily subscribe to it. ETEnergyworld.com shall not be responsible for any damage caused to any person/organization directly or indirectly.

References

1. https://www.eia.gov/outlooks/steo/report/prices.php. Accessed 27 March 2020.
2. https://www.forbes.com/sites/uhenergy/2020/03/22/lower-for-longer-covid-19s-impact-on-crude-oil-and-refined-products/#8ae7d382fe83. Accessed 27 March 2020.
3. https://seekingalpha.com/article/4333929-oil-price-might-go-negative-bullish-for-wti. Accessed 27 March 2020.

4. https://investorcenter.slb.com/static-files/60c804db-550e-4fca-a6ae-099d61940e51. Accessed 27 March 2020.
5. https://investorcenter.slb.com/static-files/02610827-ca39-4016-94e1-e3bbdf19ed8f. Accessed 27 March 2020.
6. https://www.aogr.com/web-exclusives/us-rig-count/2020. Accessed 27 March 2020.

Millennials and COVID-19 15

Benjamin Hidalgo[a], Gerald Marín-García[b], Edwin Wu[c], and Allyson Hidalgo[d]

[a]Health Science, Phoenix, AZ, United States, [b]Critical Care-Emergency Medicine Physician, VA Caribbean Healthcare System, San Juan, Puerto Rico, [c]Intensive Care Solutions, Baptist Hospital, Miami, FL, United States, [d]Biochemistry, Arizona State University, Phoenix, AZ, United States

Personal experience, conversations with a post-COVID-19 patient, and some questions to think about

I'm writing this chapter in the month of June. Surprisingly, the quarantine has been lifted, and the economy is now "reopened." There have been protests against the quarantine, and now, there are protests against the police that have turned to riots. Grocery stores all require sanitized carts; we're using bottles of hand sanitizer after touching anything from gas station pumps, apartment lobby keypads, and elevator buttons. As I'm taking my younger sister grocery shopping with me, I see that the Sprouts Farmers Market we frequent has boarded up all its windows and doors in precaution against looters. I turn to her and say "Wow, we really are in an apocalypse."

Some people had stocked up on toilet paper upon hearing the first rumors of quarantine, thinking that resources would be limited. In reality, the supply chain was not affected. Others stockpiled ammunition in fears of a necessary civil war since a curfew and quarantine apparently mean martial law. And here we are now: a curfew is enforced and the National Guard's Humvees are parked at every entrance of the shopping malls, guarding them from looters. But how did we get to this point?

It seems to me that the people have been easily driven mad and we are just looking for some sense of solidarity. We're all just looking for some purpose to get behind amidst the civil unrest, the economy's uncertainty, and the pandemic's threats that made us tremble, although it seems we have forgotten about the latter. These protests against the quarantine and the police force in the United States have led to the same types of mass gatherings we had worked so hard to prevent.

As I'm writing this in Tempe, Arizona, I'm reading news that Arizona's infection rate is now more than three times higher than that of New York State. There have been more than 4400 new cases reported in the past 72 h. Arizona is now the number 1 state for coronavirus disease (COVID) cases, and it's no surprise to me at all. Apart from these mass gatherings, all the bars are now open. I've seen pictures and videos on friends' social media, and it really seems like everything is back to "normal." It seems to me that our leaders are just "winging it." It's almost simply up to us to educate ourselves and propagate that information to our peers, since we lack so much guidance. I'm not sure that we can just expect the masses to take responsibility and be the ones to flatten the curve. If our leaders don't set the example, if they don't model the way, what are we expected to do? Clearly, we need more educated leadership. We need more competent leaders versed in these matters. It's so concerning to me, and nearly obvious that there will definitely be a second wave, considering this is such a highly infectious virus.

I'm working on a Master's Degree of Healthcare Management at the University of Arizona and I hope that what I'm working toward will be a stepping stone to becoming a leader in my field. I hope I can be a part of efforts to educate the masses, perhaps advise those in political positions and perhaps play an important role in managing aspects of national and even global health, as it is clearly necessary in times like these. I currently work as a nursing assistant, and when I'm in the hospital, I'm required to don full personal protective equipment: mask, goggles, apron, double gloves, and boot covers, just to come into brief contact with a post-COVID patient. The term "post-COVID" means that he/she has had the virus in the past and is now awaiting a confirmation of a negative test result. All this, for just a potential exposure to COVID 2019 (COVID-19), and what we have on the polar opposite side of the coin are crowded bars, clubs, restaurants, and mass gatherings.

I've been exposed to COVID-19 and have contracted the virus unfortunately as well. When I first suspected my infection, I had a shift at work the following morning. I had some symptoms like a runny nose, chills, sore throat, and what I consider the cardinal two: complete loss of taste and smell. I couldn't smell the coffee I was drinking, or taste the cumin in my chicken. I knew my team needed me. I knew the consequences of not being on the hospital floor and forcing them to be understaffed. I knew that without my contribution, they would struggle. It was a difficult decision, but my conscience forced me to make the choice I did of calling off work that day. I couldn't go to work and put the lives of my patients at risk. I didn't know if I had the virus, but I wasn't going to put the lives of the people I'm supposed to care for in danger simply due to my negligence. I phoned in to the hospital, called off my shift, and reported my possible infection. I know they really wanted me there. Apparently with a flu, you're not considered contagious unless you actively have a fever. If I didn't have a fever, I would have been "cleared" and considered fine to work. I was asked if I had one, and I lied saying yes, because I knew that even asymptomatic individuals could carry and pass on the virus.

The charge nurse told me I needed to get tested to confirm my exposure immediately, and that I would need a negative test result in order to return. That sounded to me like very effective protocol. I scheduled a test for the next day, and headed to bed. The next day, I woke up feeling extreme fatigue, muscle aches, and chills. I headed to the testing site and awaited my results, which I was informed would take another 2–5 days. Thankfully, they were prompt, and I received a result in 2 days: I was positive for COVID-19. I followed the recommended procedure by the Centers for Disease Control and Prevention (CDC) and stayed at home for the following 14 days. I was aware that the incubation period for the virus, or the time from exposure to symptom onset could have been anywhere from 3 to 6 days, so I wasn't sure of when I might have contracted it. I tested again 8 days from my positive result and received a second positive.

I was feeling ok by this time, hoping for that negative result. I enjoy my work, and I'm sure no one likes being locked up in the house all day, so I was a little bit let down, but I had to follow through with my responsibility. If I ventured out of the house I may not be directly putting those I have contact with at risk, but I could be endangering the lives of their relatives, or other people they encounter. I had planned ahead from the beginning of the outbreak anyway. Before there was a mandatory lockdown, I purchased enough canned food and other items with a long shelf life to last me 3 weeks, so I wasn't really in need of anything. I'm lucky to have people looking out for me as well. Some were very good friends, and everyone in my family called to check up on my condition. They offered to bring me anything I needed, which I really appreciated. Thankfully, my parents had already prepared my sister and I for the potential outbreak by sending us Sudafed and Sudagrip, which helped with the fever and chills, so I wasn't in any need of medications either. Instead I offered my family some of my medication in case they were ever infected. The CFO and staff managers of the hospital I work at sent me text messages from their personal phones to ask how I was doing and if there was anything I needed. The gesture really meant a lot to me because it is reinforced the way I felt about the culture in the environment I work in. It's a small hospital, and we're all members of a health-care team. It taught me that the team effort to care for others goes beyond just the workplace.

I received another call from the charge nurse at the hospital on Friday of the second week of my self-quarantine. I was asked a couple of questions about my symptoms, and if I had a fever. I didn't have a fever and was told that as long as I had been fever-free for at least 3 days, I could be cleared and be able to return to work. I was surprised by this and was on board with it. I would have liked to receive a negative result prior to returning to work, but I could only do so much, right? If those in management say that it is okay for me to go back, then I maybe I should be ok. I did what I could, and they're the medical professionals after all. I may not necessarily agree with the situation but what more can I do? I would have fulfilled the 14 days of quarantine from the first day of my positive result by the time of my upcoming shift, according to CDC guidelines, so in the end, I did my part after all, and followed the guidelines I was supposed to. I said I was in agreement and was scheduled to work on Sunday, 3 days from the time of that phone call.

The very next day, I felt chills and muscle aches once more. My first fever actually started that night. It didn't make any sense to me. How could I be getting a fever this late into the infection? I didn't say anything to my team, hoping for the best the following day, but nothing changed. I still had the same symptoms, and this time they came with even more fatigue. I called in sick to work again. Another day passed and I noticed a slight discomfort in my throat. It felt as if I had swallowed something sharp, and it had scratched my esophagus on the way down. The pain was unbearable the following day. It hurt so much to swallow my own saliva. I was drooling and spitting from how much I was avoiding having to swallow. My doctor told me that I had contracted a throat infection by opportunistic bacteria possibly as a sequela due to the immunosuppression of having been infected with COVID-19. This infection lasted about 5 debilitatingly painful days, during which I tested for the virus a third time, and finally received the negative result I was hoping for. I was so glad to have had a negative result before returning to work.

My case was nowhere near as severe as what some others have experienced, however. I recognize my privilege and fortune to be young, healthy, and to have no preexisting conditions during this pandemic. The hospital I work at is a rehabilitation hospital. This means that patients in the process of recovering from accidents, falls, orthopedic surgery, stroke or traumatic brain injuries, etc. come to our facility to recuperate and engage in daily physical therapy. Some of these patients who had been previously diagnosed with the virus were recovering from having been put on a ventilator. I tried to be as sensitive as possible when asking my patients about their experiences.

"If you don't mind me asking, what was your experience with COVID-19?" I asked one of my patients. He looked like he was in pretty good shape, and he was recovering well.

"What was my experience? Like what did I go through?" He asked me to clarify.

"Yes. How did you know you were infected?" I continued.

He began to explain, "I didn't know I was infected." He told me that he started having chills and muscle aches while he was at home, but he had no other symptoms. He went through a couple of days, like this before going to the hospital. "I wasn't even planning to go to the doctor at all," he confessed. "I have so much lapse in memory that I'm not exactly even sure what is a dream and what isn't. It all feels surreal to me. I'm not even sure how lucid I am here in front of you today." I gave him a look of concern as I kneeled in front of him to place anti-embolic stockings on his legs. "When I was at home I started having a slight cough. It was nothing crazy, just a small itch in my throat I felt I was trying to clear it up. All I know is that night when I went to bed I was having trouble breathing, and my wife suggested that we'd best go to the hospital before my condition got any worse." I took a seat after having put his socks on and continued listening. "The next thing I remember is that I was seated in the emergency room. They told me I fainted there, and my next memory after that is being in a hospital bed while the paramedic asked me to sign some things. I wasn't even sure what I was signing, and there I have another lapse in memory. I don't know if this is the next day, or the same day, the next week or whatever; I just remember the doctors coming in and explaining the necessity for me to be put on a ventilator, and asking if I was in agreement with the procedure. I simply said 'Whatever the doctor says is best.' And they asked me to remove my ring so that the swelling in my hands wouldn't cause me to lose a finger. I handed him my wedding ring, and that's the last thing I remember. I don't know how long I was under, and the next thing I know, I was awake again in the hospital and the next day they transferred me here."

Due to the lack of oxygen, he suffered of neuronal and permanent lung damage. This is what was causing his lapses in memory, and was affecting his level of alertness and orientation. He was very weak upon standing. His physical therapists explained to me that they weren't certain he'd be able to walk without an assistive device again. I know he's lucky to be alive. I see patients in every shift that I consider fortunate. Some of them have to relearn how to use their entire bodies all over again because they've lost motor function in their arms and legs due to the lack of oxygen to their brains. Many haven't been so fortunate and have lost their lives. Friends and family of mine have lost loved ones to this virus, and I'm grateful that the borders back home in Belize are closed. I give thanks to God for that every day. My father, who lives there, is receiving chemotherapy so this places him at risk.

As a health-care worker who constantly sees and hears cases like these, I understand the frustration that comes with this pandemic. There are human lives at stake, and there is a very demanding responsibility to do the best you can and play your part, but there are other consequences as well. Economists say, for example, that more than 40% of all job losses due to this pandemic are now permanent. Unemployment was perhaps at all-time lows before this pandemic, around 3.6%. Now, on the other hand, it could be anywhere from 10% to 25%. Experts are now linking unemployment in the United States to a death toll, explaining that every one percentage point increase could be equivalent to 40,000 deaths. With a rate of 10%–25%, I'm frightened to even do the math. The bitter truth is that this pandemic could have more consequences than those directly caused by the becoming infected with the virus itself.

Perhaps our leaders may be making the best decision after all. Are they? I truly want to believe that they are, but we are being faced such a difficult dilemma. Maybe this pandemic could have been handled differently from the start. Maybe it is too late now to remedy the problems we now have in front of us. If we take a look at the rates of infection in other countries, we can clearly see downtrends. Many countries like France, Spain, and even Italy which was once a "coronavirus hotspot" are now well under control. New Zealand did an excellent job of containing the infection rate. When we look at the United States, however, and it's clear that we didn't do a lot of things right.

Infection rates are rising even higher than the initial spike. I'm disappointed because it truly seems to me as if there is almost like a childish blame game being played by our leaders. Whether China underreported its cases or not, and whether they are responsible for a global outbreak because of their inability shut down international flights, shouldn't matter. The problems we face should not be about whose fault they are; are we really going to wager lives here and play blame games? Are we performing human sacrifice simply to make a point? I understand that the laws of power are important, but where are our ethics?

I'm hearing news now, that Belize is opening its borders on August 15, and yes, Americans are welcome... Is it not our responsibility now not to continue to spread the virus to countries that rely so much on us? If China is responsible after all, it shouldn't matter. Why don't we do what we can to contain the problem, and then seek some form of accountability? Why must we play this spiteful game as if we're saying to the world, "if they won't take accountability, we won't either"? We're simply showing that we're no better. France is now banning U.S. passports from entry to the country, and this is for a good reason. How do our actions look to the rest of the world? What impact on international relations could this have for the United States?

There's one more thing I want us to think about before I conclude. I understand that people don't like being told what to do. Perhaps we need a different approach. Who said a pandemic was going to be easy? There will always be conflict, no matter what decisions are made. If you ride the donkey into the city, people say you're being abusive to the poor animal. If you don't, they call you a fool for not utilizing it. The moral of *The Man, the Boy, and the Donkey* fable is that you can't please everyone. If we're going to "reopen the economy," then so be it. I'm not saying I agree with that decision at all, but the truth is that no one really has the solid answers for handling this situation. There were no previous protocols in recorded history for a situation like this. Frankly, I think the United States did a terrible job when we were expected to be the leaders to this side of the globe. As for what can be done now, I do think, however, that more can be done to get our people on board with the decisions being made, or at least we need more education and transparent communication between our leaders and our people.

It's a nuisance that people think you're infringing their rights of freedom simply by telling them to wear a mask, for example. At first, I didn't understand the cause for such resistance. It's not such a hard price to pay for some sort of freedom to roam outside and carry on as if we're not in the middle of a pandemic. In many Asian countries, people wear a mask when they have the flu or even just a cold, simply to do their best not to contaminate surfaces when coughing or sneezing, since the droplet particles will stick to surfaces. There is a culture of collectivism rather than the individualism we see here. Do we really lack the culture in this country to be considerate of others?

Admittedly, there could be some solid evidence that reusing a surgical mask could harbor mold or cause other problems. It is designed to be worn in a sterile environment after all. Wearing them outside in the dust with our constant humid breath behind them is not what they're designed for, and yes, an N95 mask only filters air coming in, and not the air coming out. This is because it is vented to expel the air straight out of the mask without filtration, so it would defeat the purposed of wearing a mask in order to protect others from yourself. It is designed to be worn in contaminated environments, so there is no need to filter the breath of the person donning it. There is also the argument that cloth masks don't even filter anything. In fact, these humid barriers could become mildew ridden overnight.

Okay, I get it. There is resistance. There are potentially valid points being raised, but please, let's do some more research. The data supporting the donning of masks we've all seen on social media probably doesn't account for the things I've stated above. But what is the alternative? Are we really going to suggest that it's better that we don't wear a mask at all? A healthy individual donning a mask is significantly lowering their risk of contracting the virus. The positive effect on transmission rates is even further increased when a carrier of the virus or infected person dons a mask. Now, if everyone wears one and the rate of transmission from carriers to healthy individuals is even lower. Instead of being so combative and resistant to do anything we're told, why can we not just follow through at least with that? If there's really so much concern over the masks like the arguments above then there are simple solutions. Let's change the disposable surgical masks daily. Let's not wear N95, and I assumed everyone was already doing so, but how about we wash out cloth masks daily? Most importantly, however, how about we just wear them? Is this really so hard to do or must we really behave like rebellious teenagers?

There will always be people who are drawn to conspiracy theories. Let's face it. I have friends that I feel bad for, who eat these sorts of things up. They're constantly complaining about social media not allowing them to propagate false information because their posts have been "fact checked." Their accounts get flagged, and their response to this is, "they are censoring us."

I don't agree, but I can understand their points of view and their frustrations. Maybe we shouldn't be removing their posts, "infringing their freedom of speech," but how do you pull people out of that line of thinking and get them to just face the scientific facts? Maybe we shouldn't censor them because in so doing, we may only pushing them to hold on to these ideas more strongly. They say this virus could have been engineered in a laboratory somewhere and that it has something to do with 5G towers. Perhaps COVID-19 isn't even real, and "the media" is really just distracting us from other things going on behind the scenes. I get it. Those in power will do anything to keep the current systems in place in order to sustain that power. There will always be distractions for the masses while more sinister things take place in the background. There might never be true transparency in the world we live in, but the message all of this communicates to me is that people simply don't trust their leaders. Given history of our country, frankly, I don't blame them.

I do want to, however, do what I can to lay these concerns to rest. I hope there are readers who can change their minds, or maybe you, the reader, can use the following thought exercise to try to knock someone out of those "conspiracy theorist" lines of thinking. Sometimes what I really want to ask these people are: "So you don't trust the government thinking that they could be using surgical masks to control us? We are literally carrying tracking devices in our pockets everywhere we go. The National Security Agency possibly has a record of every message or phone conversation you've had for the past 10 years. We're all forced to register our property and pay taxes under a social security number given to us at birth for the sole purpose of keeping track of our contributions to society. You have a social security number, a driver's license number, a passport number, license plate number, and house number. They know everything about us, and already have the power to control us, but are we really going to believe they're using the masks, of all things, to control us?"

Millennials and the COVID-19 pandemic
Perspective from an avid trainee

Uncertainty was the main driver of this fear. There were no established protocols. We were extrapolating data from previous pandemics and other organisms. At this point, we only knew that it had a genetic resemblance to the severe acute respiratory syndrome virus. However, this was not enough as we did not know about its disease course, infectivity, virulence, and so forth. While we wanted to fight this virus and save people's lives; how were we going to protect ourselves and our families? Is it a droplet isolation organism? Is it an airborne disease? Too many questions were still unanswered.

As trainees, we had teachers and mentors who were willing to guide us. However, just like everyone else, they were victims of the lack of facts. Slowly, leaders emerged. Attending physicians and co-fellows started integrating different protocols and adapting them to our capabilities. They were teaching us how to use personal protective equipment appropriately prior to evaluating a COVID-19 patient. Taking video of those training activities so we could teach ancillary staff. Those leaders knew that the only way to fight this fear is by defeating the uncertainty, defeating it with knowledge.

We thought we were making a lot of progress in getting prepared. And indeed, we were. However, our reality was more like that old cliché say: "When I had all the answers, the questions changed". Impotency was added to the fear as a worldwide shortage in personal protective equipment was booming. News about the lack of mechanical ventilators in New York was developing. We were not in that position, but by that time, we knew we could not underestimate COVID-19. The mere possibility of having to decide who gets a mechanical ventilator and who dies, still to this day gives me goosebumps.

It finally happened, we got out first confirmed COVID-19 patient. You could sense the tension, the fear on the unit. The fear of what was once unknown and distant, now is present and real. I love my job. I love what I do. Like most people in my generation, we think about work-life integration instead of work-life balance. We think we need to have fun while we work rather than after. The moment that patient arrived at the unit, everyone lost their smile. But, since we are devoted to taking care of sick people, we ignored that we were not having fun and did our job. Physicians, pharmacists, nurses, respiratory therapists, and clerical and maintenance workers; everyone did their best to try to hide their emotions and started taking care of the patient. One patient quickly became two, then three. Not everyone was strong enough, though. Some people were too afraid to work. We had critical care patients who could not receive official ultrasounds, echocardiograms, or other necessary processes. We understood that exposure needed to be minimized. But sometimes, despite our best efforts, our bedside tools were not enough. We needed a lending hand that was just not available. But then again, who could blame them. After all, we were becoming used to these patients and dealing with the fear, but they were not. They were in the same phase of uncertainty, we were several weeks prior.

We had not been hit as hard as other places. The number of sick patients who we had encountered was not elevated. However, just the mere possibility of the pandemic getting out of control in our hospital, kept us focused. We geared our efforts into studying all the COVID-19 literature, or so we thought. We tried to keep up with the copious amount of literature to provide optimal patient care. But this was unachievable. The sheer amount of literature that was coming out every day, mostly "expert" opinion, was more difficult to handle than the number of critical COVID-19 patients we had. It was exhausting. However, we had to keep trying and be the best physician we could for our patients. Everyone shimmed in. Short summaries of anything published was read. It got to a point it was so repetitive that it was frustrating.

Day in and day out, we tried our best. Fear was not such a big factor for us now. Sorrow started to takeover. It broke our hearts that people were under our care for months now. Their families were only hearing bad news and kept hanging on to those memories of their healthy loved ones. They were unable to see them. Unable to say how much they missed and loved them. We needed to evolve, do something, and use the available technology to demonstrate our empathy. We had tablets that were given to us, to facilitate consultant interaction without exposure to the COVID-19 patient. One day, an attending physician used the tablet to call the spouse of an intubated patient who was not improving. We then quickly realized how just seeing and talking to the patient, gave families some closure and strength to keep the hope alive. This "lesson" would have never been found in the literature that we were reading. After that day, that was the norm. In the afternoon, after rounds, we called one family member of every single patient on the phone. On alternate days, we took them to the room with the tablet. This was the new way of placing the hand on the back of a sad family member, the modern way of showing compassion and empathy.

As the dust settled and more information was available, the uncertainty decreased. The concept of gratifying work returned. We were smiling, enjoying once again what we were doing. The ecstasy of our COVID-19 experience was when we extubated our first patient. Every team member had a part on that success. We knew the patient was slowly reaching the goal. That morning, in rounds, the patient showed all the required signs to be extubated. We asked the patient via signals he wanted to get the tube out. At that time, the patient gave us the most strong and convincing thumbs up we had ever seen. We proceeded to extubate him. Not 5 min had passed, and we were running to get the tablet so we could surprise the spouse. As we made the call and showed the spouse what had just happened, everyone's eyes filled with tears. Tears of happiness for them and hope that this pandemic could be beaten.

COVID-19 has changed everyone's lives. We need to continue to encourage and practice prevention and lead the masses by example. Social distancing measures, hand hygiene, and wearing mask are simple things that can be done when compared to what the patients and family members have gone through. This is just beginning. We are far from been done with this virus. We cannot let our guards down. Until a vaccine is available, no major changes are likely to occur. However, once a vaccine is produced, a new challenge will arise. People might be hesitant to get it. We need to start with an aggressive campaign on how a massive vaccination program is the most viable solution. It would not be an easy task, but then again, with COVID-19 nothing has.

If we could go back in time, I wish we would not have underestimated the virulence and infectivity of this virus. For future threats, we need to prepare sooner to readily assess the capabilities and flaws in the system. But regardless, the amount of effort, camaraderie, and empathy that has resurfaced, made this a unique experience. In trying to be optimistic and looking at the "COVID-19 glass" half full, what we have faced in the last couple of months made us grow significantly as physicians and humans. As a medical trainee, I could not have asked for more.

COVID-19: Data collection and transparency among countries

16

Erwin Calgua

Research Center of Health Sciences, School of Medicine, University of San Carlos of Guatemala, Guatemala City, Guatemala

Introduction

The coronavirus disease 2019 (COVID-19) pandemic is a public health problem with extensive implications for health systems and economies around the globe. The first cases were reported as a pneumonia of unknown origin in Wuhan, China, on December 31, 2019.[1] The World Health Organization (WHO) announced through social media outlets about these cases during the first week of January, and in the same week, the agent was identified as a severe acute respiratory syndrome coronavirus 2 (SARS-CoV-2).[2] This new coronavirus showed immediately the attribute to spread efficiently to new countries and regions outside China, such as Philippines, France, Italy, Spain, and the United States.

It is important to note that the first data was collected and analyzed by local Chinese authorities where the outbreak was taking place, and the timing that took identifying the first case to the moment that they shared the information with WHO was reported as immediate, a claim that was not challenged in the first phase of the pandemic. Another interesting fact is that, in the very beginning, WHO or the scientific community did not have any doubt about the authenticity of the data being shared by Chinese officials. The data began to flow through the weekly WHO bulletins, and later, the Johns Hopkins University (JHU) developed the Coronavirus Resource Center that kept track of the coronavirus cases based largely on data provided by 188 different countries and regions of the world.[3]

As the pandemic developed, most individuals turned to the JHU resource to have a timely and reliable data of the COVID-19 cases. As of the preparation of this chapter, this resource has been the most popular (even more popular that the official site of WHO for COVID-19[4]), despite the fact that a few actually know where the data for its dashboard comes from, and even less, take the time to verify the authenticity of the source of the data used for this information, which includes media reports. For a while, this information was not challenged, but as the dynamic of the pandemic developed, questions arose about the data that were collected and about the information provided after the analysis of such data. Here is where the issue of transparency emerged, especially triggered by the reports that questioned the information provided by Chinese officials in regard to the start of the pandemic. At the same time, similar concerns were raised in other high-income countries,[5] including lower middle-income countries like Guatemala, that challenged the transparency of the data and information presented by local authorities.

With this chapter, we want the reader to have a brief overview, from the perspective of a clinical epidemiologist, of the lessons learned on two key epidemiological aspects in the process to inform authorities and society related to COVID-19 being those: (1) data collection and (2) transparency in the data.

Lessons learned about COVID-19 data collection

The WHO is the leading institution when it comes to data and information related to an epidemiological emergency.[6] For the purposes of this chapter, it is important to understand that WHO's key role is to coordinate data collection and provides information based on analysis of the data in a global context. Based on this information, technical and financial support is provided to countries around the globe. Of utmost importance is to note that WHO monitors constantly the data and information that is provided by the different countries and regions of the world.[7] Also, interesting to note is that collecting the data in a dynamic global context is both a strength and a weakness, because what WHO gains from obtaining data of authorities, losses in the quality of the data that is provided by Ministries of Health, that respond directly to the highest authorities in government who decide which data and when the data is released, something that is of key importance when making decisions in the midst of an epidemiological emergency, as the current COVID-19 pandemic.

During the first days of the COVID-19 pandemic, there were no questions, at least in the general public, about the data and information that was provided through WHO bulletins or the JHU site, especially the ones that came from China. Then, as the virus spread around the globe, data from France, Italy, Spain, and the United States emerged, and in a similar manner, there were no questions about the data and information. But things began to change as the pandemic evolved, and questions began to raise in regard to the data and information provided by China, after the concerns that were expressed by the highest authorities in the United States government.

As a response, China issued a statement which confirmed that they have followed the protocols and processes required by WHO in matters pertaining to data collection and reporting, making emphasis that they have complied with all these standards based on international agreements, in a timely manner. We must draw the attention that at this point, there were no questions from WHO or other key institutions leading to believe that the data collection and analysis provided by China or any other government around the world were flawed. However, the media and news outlets, through investigative journalist methods,[8] inquired about the authenticity of the data provided by governments and centered their attention in the question of hidden data. The investigations lead to findings such as that the first case could have been in the mid of November 2019.[9] In addition, independent investigators from Harvard

University conducted a study based on satellite pictures and online searches around the Wuhan area and reported that the first cases could have happened as early as August 2019[10]. Through these findings, we have learned two important lessons which are: first, media and news outlets play a key role in creating questions for the public opinion about the way data are obtained and how this information is communicated, and second, the importance of trust in local and global authorities about the transparency in management of data collection and generation of information, as it is mentioned in WHO fundamental guidelines on how to collect data during epidemiological emergencies.

Lessons learned about COVID-19 data transparency

Transparent is defined as being "free from pretense or deceit",[11] and it is expected that by all means, a government is committed to be obedient to the law, and even more, comply with high ethical standards in the way that manage data and communicate information to increase the benefits for the general public and avoid risk that could harm their lives. This, in short, should be the main aspects that any government should follow, so the mitigation directions issued are followed by society and in that way prevent the impact and high cost in morbidity and mortality of vulnerable populations during an epidemiological emergency.

So far, COVID-19 pandemic has been a challenge in regard to empower governments to lead the actions that could mitigate the impact of this virus in their countries. China, being a high-income country, has been questioned about the transparency of the data and information that provided to the world.[12] One of the errors they have made was the decision to control and limit the scientific information that was requested by the scientific communities[13] to understand better how SARS-CoV-2 appeared and behaved. No information could be provided without government authorization. That simple decision created a distrust in what was reported by Chinese institutions, something that has remained to date and could take time to overcome. Therefore the sole reaction of limiting the information was perhaps one of the most damaging actions of the Chinese government, and the worst part is that the media was not the only one reporting the lack of transparency from the Chinese government but also the scientific networks around the world raised their concern that Chinese scientists were coerced to not to share their data and information and even seek collaborations with scientists who wanted to understand better COVID-19 as the SARS-CoV-2 was spreading to other countries.

Unfortunately, similar attitudes were shown governments of lower middle-income countries, like Guatemala where the first case was reported on March 13. During the first month, the information provided by the Ministry of Health was openly received by media outlets, population, and scientific community, and in short, no questions were made as of the reliability and timely manner that this was received. However, as the pandemic developed, the scientific community and society had concerns about the number of COVID-19 tests that were performed. Certainly, the acquisition of tests was a very difficult and important issue to address, from the government perspective, and even more challenging was to communicate to the general public about the lack of tests around the globe[14]. Among the general public, it is a common belief that a test has been validated by the time that a pandemic starts, and just a few could understand that such is not the case in certain epidemiological emergencies as was the case for SARS-CoV-2. Societies believe that funding is enough to secure a test, and in certain way it does, but with SARS-CoV-2, the issue of having funds did not secure the possibility of having a reliable test in which the health systems could trust to identify the cases among the general population. Therefore, there was a key communication issue that needed to be addressed, which was to explain the relation that has the availability of a test and the possibility to confirm a case (no test, no data), which limits the possibility to understand how a highly infectious disease behaves from the beginning.

Another situation that happened in Guatemala was the presidential daily briefing that presented to the public the COVID-19 information. The format of such briefings was inconsistent, and there was a lack of clarity for the general public. Therefore, the Guatemalan population did not completely understand the data and even noticed when contradicted data was presented to them. Based on that, as in China, news outlets[15] in Guatemala began to search deeply into the information[16] and finally, the government acknowledged that there was a sub-registry in the data that they were providing during the briefing and error not directly related to the lack of tests, but of information that was not transferred to them, especially, in regard to the number of deaths occurring in Guatemala. What should be considered as simple situation turned out to be a key issue that has been the center of what is considered as the main driver of the lack of success in the mitigation measures implemented by the government, which was the perception of lack of transparency and fear of corruption that was reported in the media,[17] and eventually, this ended up in the distrust on government planning and decisions, which lead to an increased number of COVID-19 cases, something that has been the trend to the day that this chapter was written.

What could be implemented to improve data collection for COVID-19

If data collection is a fundamental aspect that must be defined in the beginning of an epidemiological emergency, then it is important that Ministries of Health, as the highest authorities, must clearly define the procedures that not only locally but also globally must govern the data collection and subsequent storage and analysis to provide timely and reliable information. One main limitation that exists around the globe is that there is not a universal validated tool that could be used and applied in local and international contexts to collect data with the purpose of informing in a timely manner of the cases who are identified during an epidemic crisis.

There have been efforts to develop such tools, but the initiatives have moved only to the stage of a proposal, never becoming a universal tool that could be used by

Ministries of Health. There could be many reasons that could explain why the implementation of such tools might be challenging. First, there are "political" reasons, which usually are more economical reasons, that intentionally avoid to create a collaborative environment. It has been well established that when a country faces an epidemiological emergency, the economic impact becomes the highest priority relegating the provision of adequate health services to a last place. In many ways, COVID-19 is teaching us that prioritizing the economic factors over the health will eventually lead to a more complex health problem. Hiding the data from the international scientific community, and not giving time to carefully analyze it, will eventually create a situation that will affect not only the country that was primarily affected but also the globe to a point that even commerce could stagger and deepen the economic inequalities.[18] Governments, and specifically Ministries of Health, must carefully begin to outline clear policies and plans that will guide actions during such epidemiological emergencies, and the first public health policy in epidemiological emergencies should be the one about data collecting and sharing with the international community and the general public.[19]

Technical teams at Ministries of Health must know that if there is a need to share data, an important issue should be what data must be collected. That takes us again to the universal tool that we have mentioned before. The tool selected must be developed in consensus with other governments, and a guideline with a clear process must be prepared to be used in epidemiological emergencies. It will be expected that such guidelines should be developed in consultation with the WHO, and a clear statement should be made within the United Nations in order to adopt such tool in a universal manner. There are immediate limitations in this proposal, mainly due to political distinctions among countries and regions, especially between world potencies, that ultimately have the possibility to vote and decide if they will adopt the tool and share this data in the areas where they exercise an economical and military influence (we must keep present that an epidemiological emergency as the SARS-CoV-2 pandemic is considered a national security concern for world potencies). Undoubtedly, there is a primary institution that should promote the development of such a tool and that should be the WHO; however, if we argue that today's pandemics have a heavy impact in international commerce, then another instance that should be considered to coordinate these efforts is the World Trade Organization (WTO). This second option should not be a surprise,[20] because we have argued before that at the beginning of a pandemic, the priorities of governments are usually commerce over health, and COVID-19 clearly has become a commerce problem with local and international implications.

Once the world has consented the organization from where this tool will be developed, then it is important to define what kind of data should be collected. This again should not be a difficult issue to define. A common mistake of Ministries of Health is trying to collect a vast amount of data that ends up in large quantities of bytes stored in some electronic device that is never analyzed. But this should change. As mentioned earlier, of key importance is to be able to accurately count the cases. COVID-19 was difficult in the aspect that there was no diagnosis test available, and once this was developed, such test was inaccessible for two reasons. First, because the technologies used to identify the antigen usually requires highly trained human resources and specialized equipment that is not easily available, especially in lower middle-income countries. Second, once the technology has been developed, there is the possibility that patents and licenses for such technologies are too expansive, that acquisition becomes prohibitive for countries that do not have the means to fund immediately the acquisition of such tests. This directly impacts the possibility to have accurate data (remember: no test, no data) that could be reported in a local and global context. Therefore every effort should be made toward obtaining and having the possibility to have availability and accessibility to a diagnosis test that could be applied globally, regardless of being in a high-, middle-, or lower-income country. Certainly, an economy based on free market will challenge this proposal; nevertheless, COVID-19 is teaching us that in a context where a pandemic exists in the free market around the world will be as strong as the weakest of the countries.

One important aspect also is to define the data that should be collected.[21] It is possible that the first data that must be collected will be the cases confirmed by an accurate diagnostic test. The second data that should be obtained is the swabs performed.[22] Interestingly, most of the countries report the number of positive cases per day; however, this might be accurate for high-income countries where there is the technology readily available and in a short amount of time the results are available, but it is difficult to find such situations in a lower middle-income countries. Guatemala's experience was that in some cases it took 8 days to report the test result. So, the fact that this was presented as positive in a given date, which did not reflect the exact moment of when the case was happening, giving an inaccurate picture of the situation in real time.[23] Is in that regard that it would be preferable to report the number of positive cases based on the daily swabs than the daily performed diagnosis.

The third data will be the number of deaths related to COVID-19, which is another important and challenging data that must be collected and reported. The challenge of this data is that it also needs to have a positive test for the diagnosis; however, it would be even better if the death could be also confirmed with an autopsy. But, the fact that most health services lack a test at the beginning of the pandemic, and it is not readily available for a long time, as previously stated, it might be difficult for countries to have a positive test on one end. On the other end, most health services, once the patient dies, immediately proceed to bury the cadaver without an autopsy. The lack of an autopsy limits the possibility to better understand the viral action in all the systems that comprise the human body. What would be better and should be suggested, is to conduct autopsies of the cases[24] and report the number of autopsies that finally confirms that the death was directly related to COVID-19.[25] Other mandatory data must be collected, like demographic data from the patient, length of hospitalization, etc. These suggestions of data that could be collected have the potential to inform more than a vast number of pages with information that none reads or finds practical use in order to inform decisions at all levels of public health and clinical settings.

In a global context, it would be suggested to have few data that could be shared immediately to a central organization that could collect timely and reliable data from all Ministries of Health around the world and have an accurate image of the global situation in a given epidemiological emergency.

What could be implemented to improve data transparency for COVID-19

Given the sensitive nature of the data and information that is generated during an epidemiological emergency (something that was previously stated), one of the most important challenges is how to manage this information once it reaches the government authorities. The decision on how and when information will be released to the general public ends up at the top level of a government, usually the President or Prime Minister. The decision will be driven by many factors, overall, the economic impact that could have the release of such information to the public. However, governments need to rethink and define immediately laws and policies based on firm moral grounds that clearly state that, under an epidemiological emergency, key data will be collected and shared through a central organization and that will finally create the possibility to report at least the above-mentioned indicators.

As of today, there are guidelines, mostly weak, in regard on how to proceed with providing the information to the entities that coordinate the global efforts of a pandemic, but this has not been reinforced. Undoubtedly, there is need that countries agree to develop such laws and policies within their countries, and after passing these laws locally, this must be communicated to a centralized organization body and abide by such laws and policies to move forward and begin to have a universal system that collects such data and communicates such data around the globe.

An important aspect of all this is that transparency is deeply rooted in moral arguments more than legal. The implications to abide such laws and policies will be of key importance in order to develop trust in the general public, and again, trust is of key importance when managing an epidemic crisis. The teams who will need to discuss the laws and policies must write them based on firm arguments that will stand even in the most difficult and perilous situations. COVID-19 has shown us how the lack of transparency can undermine any effort directed to mitigate the effect of pandemic. Even more important, transparency could create an environment of peace instead of conflict between nations, which has been an important subject with deep effects, like the one raised by the United States and Chinese governments[26, 27] or more locally like the one in Guatemala where the lack of transparency by the government ended up in the distrust of the population and therefore the increased number of cases and unmanageable situation of the pandemics.

Conclusion

In conclusion, data collection and transparency are two important topics closely related with strong impact in the appropriate management of an epidemiological emergency. COVID-19 has thought us globally and locally that economic impact drives the decision on how the data is obtained and what is released to the public. So far, both in high-income countries like China or low-middle–income countries like Guatemala, there is a perception that the data was flaw and inaccurate[28], and therefore, that lead to a situation of distrust that worsened the crisis. It is proposed that based on the lessons learned, that a centralized organization, whether this be WHO or WTO, collects few but substantial data that could be used for global and local decisions, data like number of positive tests, positive swabs and autopsies per day should be considered, but is not limited to this three, as there are other important demographic and clinical data that could be obtained and reported. In addition, local laws and policies related to transparency should be discussed and approved by governments in order to develop trust in the public opinion, which plays a key role in the ethical, legal, and appropriate way to manage an epidemiological emergency like the one we have experienced with COVID-19.

References

1. Archived: WHO Timeline—COVID-19. *Retrieved July 4, 2020, from*; 2020. https://www.who.int/news-room/detail/27-04-2020-who-timeline- - -covid-19.
2. WHO. *Novel coronavirus (COVID-19)*. *Retrieved July 4, 2020, from*; 2020. https://www.who.int/bulletin/online_first/COVID-19/en/.
3. COVID-19 Map - Johns Hopkins Coronavirus Resource Center. *Retrieved July 4, 2020, from*; 2020. https://coronavirus.jhu.edu/map.html.
4. WHO Coronavirus Disease (COVID-19) Dashboard. *WHO Coronavirus Disease (COVID-19) Dashboard*; 2020. Retrieved July 4, 2020, from https://covid19.who.int/?gclid=EAIaIQobChMI_LmtvIGz6gIVCgSRCh1lSgMTEAAYASABEgK96PD_BwE.
5. Should we believe the reported COVID-19 data, statistics and headlines? - Coronavirus (COVID-19) - Australia. *Retrieved July 4, 2020, from*; 2020. https://www.mondaq.com/australia/operational-impacts-and-strategy/928868/should-we-believe-the-reported-covid-19-data-statistics-and-headlines.
6. Rao C. Medical certification of cause of death for COVID-19. In: *Bulletin of the World Health Organization*. Vol. 98, Issue 5. World Health Organization; 2020. https://doi.org/10.2471/BLT.20.257600.
7. Moorthy V, Restrepo AMH, Preziosi MP, Swaminathan S. Data sharing for novel coronavirus (COVID-19). In: *Bulletin of the World Health Organization*. Vol. 98, Issue 3. World Health Organization; 2020:150. https://doi.org/10.2471/BLT.20.251561.
8. Can We Believe Any of China's Coronavirus Numbers? *Time*; 2020. Retrieved July 4, 2020, from https://time.com/5813628/china-coronavirus-statistics-wuhan/.
9. 1st known case of coronavirus traced back to November in China. *Live Science*; 2020. Retrieved July 4, 2020, from https://www.livescience.com/first-case-coronavirus-found.html.

10. Coronavirus: Fact-checking claims it might have started in August 2019. *BBC News*; 2020. Retrieved July 4, 2020, from https://www.bbc.com/news/world-asia-china-53005768.

11. Transparent Definition of Transparent by Merriam-Webster. Retrieved July 4, 2020, from (n.d.). https://www.merriam-webster.com/dictionary/transparent.

12. Western calls for greater Chinese transparency on the coronavirus reflect a clash of culture. *South China Morning Post*; 2020. Retrieved July 4, 2020, from https://www.scmp.com/comment/opinion/article/3081931/western-calls-greater-chinese-transparency-coronavirus-reflect.

13. COVID-19 research checks could deter global collaboration. *Retrieved July 4, 2020, from*; 2020. https://www.universityworldnews.com/post.php?story=20200415141352492.

14. Why America's coronavirus testing problem is so difficult to solve. *Vox*; 2020. Retrieved July 4, 2020, from https://www.vox.com/recode/2020/4/24/21229774/coronavirus-covid-19-testing-social-distancing.

15. China says it backs WHO in tracing COVID-19, denounces U.S. "lies". *Reuters*; 2020. Retrieved July 4, 2020, from https://www.reuters.com/article/us-health-coronavirus-china/china-says-it-backs-who-in-tracing-covid-19-denounces-u-s-lies-idUSKBN22J10G.

16. Coronavirus in Guatemala: 38 deaths per covid-19 had not been recorded due to a "technical failure". *Free Press*; 2020. Retrieved July 4, 2020, from https://www.prensalibre.com/guatemala/comunitario/coronavirus-en-guatemala-38-fallecidos-por-covid-19-no-habian-sido-registrados-debido-a-una-falla-tecnica/.

17. Corruption and the Coronavirus. *News*; 2020. Transparency.org. Retrieved July 4, 2020, from https://www.transparency.org/en/news/corruption-and-the-coronavirus#.

18. Ludovic J, Bourdin S, Nadou F, Noiret G. Economic globalization and the COVID-19 pandemic: global spread and inequalities. *Bull World Health Organ*. 2020. https://doi.org/10.2471/BLT.20.261099. E-pub (April).

19. Goldacre B, Harrison S, Mahtani KR, Heneghan C. *WHO consultation on Data and Results Sharing During Public Health Emergencies. Background Briefing. Sep 2015 Centre for Evidence-Based Medicine Background Briefing: WHO Consultation on Data and Results Sharing During Public Health Emergencies Background Briefing for WHO consultation on Data and Results Sharing During Public Health Emergencies*; 2015.

20. WTO - WHO coordinate action on COVID-19 pandemic - Caribbean News Global. Retrieved July 4, 2020, from. (n.d.) https://www.caribbeannewsglobal.com/wto-who-coordinate-action-on-covid-19-pandemic/.

21. Department of Health. *7.5 What data should be collected during the early stages of a pandemic?*; 2006. Retrieved July 4, 2020, from https://www1.health.gov.au/internet/publications/publishing.nsf/Content/mathematical-models~mathematical-models-discussion.htm~mathematical-models-7.5.htm.

22. Better COVID-19 data without universal testing ImmunizationEconomics.org. (2020). Retrieved July 4, 2020, from http://immunizationeconomics.org/recent-activity/2020/4/20/better-covid-19-infection-data-without-universal-testing.

23. London JW. *Covid-19: Leading statistician slams UK's reporting of swab tests as "travesty of science"*; 2020. https://doi.org/10.1136/bmj.m1664.

24. Salerno M, Sessa F, Piscopo A, et al. No autopsies on COVID-19 deaths: a missed opportunity and the lockdown of science. *J Clin Med*. 2020;9(5):1472. https://doi.org/10.3390/jcm9051472.

25. Analysis of COVID-19 autopsies reveals many new details about this disease. (n.d.). Retrieved July 4, 2020, from https://medicalxpress.com/news/2020-05-analysis-covid-autopsies-reveals-disease.html.

26. Trump claims to have evidence coronavirus started in Chinese lab but offers no details. *US news | The Guardian*; 2020. Retrieved July 4, 2020, from https://www.theguardian.com/us-news/2020/apr/30/donald-trump-coronavirus-chinese-lab-claim.

27. US urges China's "full transparency" on COVID-19. *Retrieved July 4, 2020, from*; 2020. https://www.aa.com.tr/en/americas/us-urges-china-s-full-transparency-on-covid-19/1806425.

28. They report constant discrepancies in COVID-19 information. *The Hour*; 2020. Retrieved July 4, 2020, from https://lahora.gt/senalan-discrepancias-constantes-en-informacion-de-covid-19/.

Brazilian battle against COVID-19

17

Fernando Suparregui Dias[a], Regis Goulart Rosa[b], and Ciro Leite Mendes[c,d]

[a]*Head Critical Care Department, Hospital do Circulo, Caxias do Sul, RS, Brazil* [b]*Intensive Care Unit and Research Projects Office, Hospital Moinhos de Vento, Porto Alegre, RS, Brazil* [c]*Head Intensive Care Unit, Hospital Lauro Wanderley, Universidade Federal da Paraíba, João Pessoa, PB, Brazil* [d]*Head Intensive Care Unit, Hospital Nossa Senhora das Neves, João Pessoa, PB, Brazil*

When and how did the severe acute respiratory syndrome coronavirus 2 pandemic begin in Brazil?

After the devastating effects of severe acute respiratory syndrome coronavirus 2 (SARS-CoV-2) in China, European countries, and the United States, the first case of coronavirus disease 2019 (COVID-19) in Brazil was registered on February 26, 2020, in São Paulo city. The patient was a male subject who returned from a trip to Italy and tested positive to SARS-CoV-2. In February 27, 2020, the Brazilian government informed that 20 suspect cases were monitored, from whom 12 have returned from Italy. In the same day, there were 132 suspected cases in 15 states, 85 of them were in the state of São Paulo.[1] On February 3, 2020, the Brazilian Ministry of Health declared a state of emergency due to the COVID-19 pandemic based on information on SARS cases notified to the Brazilian Information System for Notification of Grievances (a legal requirement since 2009, after the influenza A [H1N1] pandemic).[2] After then, the disease spread alongside the country, reaching 1,228,114 infected patients and 54,971 deaths by June 26, 2020.[1]

Health policies to combat the COVID-19

The public health-care system in Brazil is universal, meaning that all inhabitants are covered by the Unified Health Care System (SUS). Nevertheless, around 20% of Brazilian citizens are also covered by private health insurances, mainly in major cities and among high-income people.

Some government actions to combat the COVID-19 pandemic were as follows[3]:

1. Establishment of guidelines for COVID-19 prevention and management (https://aps.saude.gov.br/ape/corona);

COVID-19 Pandemic. https://doi.org/10.1016/B978-0-323-82860-4.00002-1

2. Allocation of 200 million reals (approximately US$ 36,496,350) to support the primary health care;
3. Extension of service hours in primary health care units;
4. Increase in the number of health-care professionals available;
5. Distribution of approximately 22 million of COVID-19 tests;
6. Implementation of a tele-system (Tele-SUS) to track back, diagnosis, and monitor patients with flu-like symptoms and COVID-19;
7. Implementation of telehealth guidance (Tele-UTI) for severe and critical cases of COVID-19;
8. Provision of a telemedicine platform for multiprofessional care; and
9. Teleconsulting with psychiatrist and psychologists.

Despite all these important measures, Brazil is facing many difficulties during the COVID-19 pandemic, mainly related to the pressure for flexibilization of social isolation, lack of medical equipment and supplies such as personal protective equipment (PPE) and mechanical ventilators, and a low availability of hospital bed and trained professionals to manage severe ill COVID-19 patients, especially in the intensive care unit (ICU).

A big concern from the Brazilian government was related to the economic impact of social isolation. In this sense, many government actions were taken in order to reopen the economy even before the peak of COVID-19 infections has been reached, sometimes ignoring the recommendations of health authorities such as the World Health Organization. Additionally, some government recommendations (e.g., hydroxychloroquine/chloroquine use) were not supported by the best available evidence, leading to doubts among health-care professionals at the front line and provoking treatment variability.

Nongovernmental initiatives were also important to combat the COVID-19 pandemic. Notably, the Epimed Solutions, a health company that collects data on health quality indicators from public and private hospitals, created a robust database including patients with SARS-CoV-2.[4] This information has been useful to identify risk areas, profile of susceptible people, resource use, outcomes, and benchmarking. Also, a partnership with the Brazilian Society of Intensive Care, the Brazilian Society of Infectious Diseases, and the Brazilian Society of Pneumology and Tisiology published rapid guidelines based on best available evidence using the GRADE system for the pharmacological treatment of COVID-19. These recommendations have been endorsed by multiple health-care professional societies and adopted in many public and private health-care contexts.

SARS-CoV-2 epidemiology in Brazil

Seventeen days went through from the first confirmed case of COVID-19, on February 26, 2020 to the 100th case. The time frames between the 100th and the 1000th, and between the 1000th and the 10,000th confirmed cases were 7 and

14 days, respectively.[5] All the Brazilian states have reported deaths related to the COVID-19. Currently, the epicenter of SARS-CoV-2 pandemic is located in São Paulo city and Rio de Janeiro. Also, cities in the North and Northeast, such as Manaus and Fortaleza, have been highly affected by the COVID-19 pandemic. In São Paulo and Rio de Janeiro, health authorities created new hospitals to attend COVID-19 patients. However, even with these measures, both public and private health-care systems are still fighting to keep ICU occupancy below 90%. Unfortunately, there was a delay to conclude COVID-19 hospitals in Rio de Janeiro, leading the public health-care system to a state of emergency. This scenario is also worrisome in North and Northeast states. Along with ICU bed scarcity, the lack of qualified health-care professionals, PPE, mechanical ventilators, and medications are challenging the quality of care provided to COVID-19 patients. In the South, the scenario seems to be less dramatic, without significant problems in bed shortage, professionals, and ICU resources. However, this context might reflect the smaller number of cases in comparison to the other geopolitical regions.

Resources and outcomes: How to solve this equation

The resource scarcity is a great challenge in Brazil. Due to lack of tests to confirm suspected cases, all patients are not being tested, prioritizing the most severe cases and high-risk groups. Unfortunately, this strategy leads to underreporting of affected patients and deaths caused by SARS-CoV-2 and biased conclusions regarding possible risks and prognostic factors.[5]

The peak of the incidence of COVID-19 seems to have already been overcome in several capitals of Brazil, which allows to partially analyze the Brazilian experience from what happened in these cities and regions. Cities as Manaus, as well as Fortaleza and Belém, just to name a few, experienced the collapse of their health systems, characterized mainly, but not exclusively, by the deficit of ICU beds. Some states, such as Paraíba, adopted social distancing early during the pandemic, which gave them time to provide infrastructure resources, but not specialized staff, which became a major limitation in providing appropriate care to critically ill patients.

Besides, even with a centralized state regulation of beds to patients with COVID-19, health-care managers were unable to promote an adequate integration, notably between the state and municipal health sectors, and this lack of integration may have contributed to a lower efficiency of COVID-19 management.

This scenario seems to have been the rule in most Brazilian states. Even where minimally adequate contingency plans were established, the lack of specialized human resources was added to problems in supply of medical materials, such as essential drugs for the management of critically ill patients, such as sedatives, neuromuscular blockers, and PPE for health professionals, which were forced, for example, to reuse N95 masks for several shifts on duty in some hospitals. The excessive demand resulting from the increasing number of severe and critical cases of COVID-19, in addition to the illness or contagion of the health professionals themselves, led the health-care institutions to hire human resources with little or no qualification. Until June 10, 2020, there was 18,354 nurses infected with SARS-CoV-2, and 182 had died, showing that in Brazil there is a critical loss of professionals caring patients with COVID-19.[6] The result could not be other than a greater proportion of unfavorable clinical outcomes, especially for cases in which recovery would depend fundamentally on specialized care.

The quality of care, despite having suffered a negative impact, proved to be acceptable so far in the face of such an adverse scenario. In a cohort of 219 patients who were admitted consecutively to an ICU intended for exclusive care of victims of COVID-19 between March and May 2020, the outcomes were reasonable despite worsening of efficiency indicators. The average age of patients was 72 years, the average length of stay in the ICU was 6.48 days, and the mortality rate was 19.72% for an average simplified acute physiology score 3 (SAPS 3) of 53.4. The standardized mortality rate was 0.8. In the year prior to the pandemic (2019), the same unit admitted 1100 patients with a mean age of 71 years, an average length of stay of 5.1 days, a mortality rate of 14.03% for an average SAPS 3 of 61.27, and standardized mortality rate of 0.49.[4] The reasons for this performance drop, in this specific center, fall on the exacerbated demand at the peak of the pandemic coupled with the need to hire nonspecialist professionals or with little experience to compose the ICU staff.

In some regions, regulatory authorities adopted criteria for admission in the ICU, in case of lack of ICU beds.[7] These recommendations intended to assist physicians in the decision-making process for ICU admission, taking into account the ethical principles of distributive justice, nonmaleficence, and respect for the autonomy and dignity of patients (Table 1).

Table 1 Guidelines for ICU admission criteria in Rio Grande do Sul, Brazil.

Priority	Criteria	Clinical aspects
Red	1	COVID-19 diagnostic criteria or high suspicion, attended in service without ICU facility, without other disease that limited prognosis before the pandemic
Orange	2	COVID-19 diagnostic criteria or high suspicion, attended in service with ICU facility crowded without other disease that limited prognosis before the pandemic
Yellow	3	COVID-19 diagnostic criteria or high suspicion, attended in service with ICU facility but indication to transfer to another more complex unit, without other disease that limited prognosis before the pandemic
Green	4	COVID-19 diagnostic criteria or high suspicion, attended in service without ICU facility, with other disease that limited prognosis before the pandemic
Blue	5	COVID-19 diagnostic criteria or high suspicion, attended in service with ICU facility, with other disease that limited prognosis before the pandemic

Lastly, in Brazil, both government and medical regulatory agencies are working together to allow the safe use of telemedicine and telehealth. Since these strategies of care can reduce, at the same time, inequities related to health access in remote and low resource areas and the risk of infection of both patients and health-care professionals, their implementation became a health priority with the COVID-19 pandemic.[5]

Opportunities for research

The SARS-CoV-2 affected all health systems in the world. The high mortality rates as well as the social and economic impact of COVID-19 pandemic impulsed research for specific SARS-CoV-2 treatments. In Brazil, some investigational initiatives are trying to contribute to the current evidence. Recently, chloroquine was tested in a randomized trial in a small group of patients from Manaus. There was a comparison between low- and high-dose regimen, and the results suggested that higher chloroquine doses are detrimental.[8] Additionally, the coalition COVID-19 Brazil initiative is currently conducting six randomized clinical trials to assess the impact of treatment candidates (e.g., hydroxychloroquine alone or in combination with azithromycin [NCT04322123, NCT04321278, RBR-3cbs3w], dexamethasone [NCT04327401], tocilizumab [NCT04403685], and anticoagulant therapy [NCT04394377] on clinical outcomes of COVID-19 patients. Notably, this initiative also includes a large follow-up study which aims to assess predictors of long-term quality of life and patient-centered outcomes among survivors of hospitalization due to COVID-19 [NCT04376658]). Probably, these results will contribute for a better understanding of COVID-19 treatment response and the impact of SARS-CoV-2 infection on patient-centered outcome in low- and middle-income settings. Another area of hope comes from the participation of 2000 Brazilian volunteers in the development of a vaccine trial, conducted by the University of Oxford, United Kingdom. This contribution should help the health organizations to manage the pandemics and stop its progression worldwide.

Lessons for the future

It is surprising and worrisome that in the 21st century, each country handled the situation according to their possibilities and resources with few global initiatives focused on quality of care and collaboration. On the other hand, despite all adversities of the situation, a lot of lessons might be learned. In Brazil in particular there are some points for evaluation: First, the governors should be acting collaboratively during a pandemic. The establishment of an effective network of collaboration between federal, state, and municipal instances across all levels of care would reduce inequalities by increasing availability of resources and improve efficiency while promoting an organized care according to the patient needs.

Second, the adoption of evidence-based practices during a pandemic should be part of the health policies of both public and private health-care systems. By supporting interventions of proven benefit or discouraging interventions that are ineffective or potential harmful, incorporating evidence into health-care practice is recognized as an essential requirement for the optimal and cost-effective care of patients.

Third, a national plan for increasing the number of ICU professionals is needed. Career development, better remuneration, and prevention of burnout are important topics to be optimized to allow a sustainable increase in the number of qualified ICU professionals in Brazil. Safer work conditions with appropriate PPE are also needed, given the high number of health-care professionals infected by the SARS-CoV-2.

Fourth, creation of national program for catastrophes management must be prioritized by health authorities. The absence of prespecified contingency plans for serious infectious diseases epidemics is unacceptable given our recent experiences. Since 2000, at least three pandemics of viral respiratory agents occurred (i.e., H5N5 in 2004, H1N1 in 2009, and SARS-CoV-2 in 2020) with many deaths and important social and economic impact. Since most of these events are unpredictable, planning and training qualified personal and provisioning appropriate material resources are essential part of damage control measures.

Fifth, a better organization in the management of health system, both in private and mainly in public organizations, is needed. Many field hospitals and ICU beds were projected but, in some states, only few completed on time. In this sense, areas able to be transformed into hospital with ICU beds should be planned, avoiding waste of time and resources implementing critical care beds during pandemics. It seems proven that from now on, any hospital should be prepared to increase its capacity in critical care beds in a short time in catastrophes.

References

1. Coronavirus Brasil. Ministério da Saúde. Accessed in 06/25/2020, n.d.
2. Bastos LS, Niquini RP, Lana RM, et al. *Rep Public Health*. 2020;36, e00070120.
3. Harzheim E, Martins C, Wollmann L, et al. Federal actions to support and strengthen local efforts to combat COVID-19: primary health care (PHC) in the driver's seat. *Ciênc Saúde Coletiva*. 2020;25:2493–2497.
4. Epimed – UTIs Brasileiras, n.d. accessed www.utisbrasileiras.com.br.
5. Caetano R, Silva AB, Guedes ACCM, et al. Challenges and opportunities for telehealth during the COVID-19 pandemic: ideas on spaces and initiatives in the Brazilian context. *Rep Public Health*. 2020;36, e00088920.
6. Rubin R, Abbasi J, Voelker R, et al. *JAMA*. 2020. published online June 12.
7. Resolução No 12, Conselho Regional de Medicina do Rio Grande do Sul. Diário Oficial da União, published in 05/29/2020, n.d.
8. Borba MGS, Almeida FF, Sampaio VS, et al. Effect of high vs low doses of choloroquine diphosphate as adjunctive therapy for patients hospitalized with severe acute respiratory syndrome coronavirus 2 (SARS-CoV-2) infection. A randomized clinical trial. *JAMA*. 2020;3, e208857.

The disproportionate burden of COVID-19 in Africa

18

Obashina Ogunbiyi

Intensive and Critical Care Society of Nigeria, Benin City, Nigeria

Introduction

The African continent is known to have a distinct epidemiological response to most of the epidemics occurring worldwide. However, it needs to be confirmed if this could be due to the tropical nature of the most African countries south of the Sahara. The burden of these various epidemics in Africa varies from that in other climates. For instance, prior to the widespread usage of vaccines against varicella in temperate, high-income countries, about 13–16 cases of varicella per 1000 population occurred annually, with children aged 1–9 years are mostly affected.[1] In those countries, over 90% of the population become infected with varicella before adolescence.[2] On the other hand, in tropical countries, including Africa, the primary infection of varicella tends to occur at a later stage in life, affecting a larger population of susceptible adults.[2]

Coronavirus disease 2019 (COVID-19) is an emerging and rapidly evolving disease which presently has attained a pandemic status, according to the World Health Organization (WHO), and it has no cure.[3] Following the above analogy, the burden of COVID-19, caused by the severe acute respiratory syndrome coronavirus 2 or novel coronavirus, in tropical Africa will be expectedly different compared to that in the Western world, made up of the "high-income countries". Despite this assumption, however, the COVID-19 disease has challenged and placed some burden on the African people with scarce resources, poor infrastructure, and unstable governments among other factors. The burden of COVID-19 also differs among the different African countries depending on the speed with which they tried to contain it, availability of testing materials, population density, clusters of population at poverty level, and health infrastructure among others. The low level of testing in some countries has made it difficult to recognize the true impact of the disease in the continent. In addition, there are associated factors of uncertain significance as the causal relationship between administration of routine BCG vaccination, in countries that have such policy, and the relatively lower COVID-19 cases and deaths compared to countries not adhered to that practice, a relation that has been studied and found to be certain, according to a multicountry level study involving 178 countries.[4]

COVID-19 Pandemic. https://doi.org/10.1016/B978-0-323-82860-4.00021-5

COVID-19: Myths and fictions

It is interesting to note that in most parts of Africa, there are some people that believe that the COVID-19 is a "scam" from the Western world to ruin our economic base or to reduce the African population. In some instances, the outbreak was followed by rumors and misinformation about the virus. This is undoubtedly impacted the efforts of containment in some countries.

One of the myths that gained ground in tropical Africa, mostly at the beginning of the pandemic, was the idea that the coronavirus would not survive the tropical weather compared to the flu, also a viral infection which presents with similar respiratory symptoms and which thrives during the cold winter season in the Western world. It was thus hoped that warmer temperatures will help in curtailing the spread of the disease. However, this was not to be, as revealed by the progressive spread in cases in the most African countries.

Another myth was the fact that drinking plenty of water was a factor in the mitigation of the virus, as water was able to dilute the viremia and flush out the virus from the body. This is premised on the social media reports of those discharged from isolation centers that they were made to drink at least 1.5 L of water daily while on admission. However, drinking water during infection with COVID-19 only helps with dehydration but does not dilute nor "flush" the virus from the body.

The art of washing hands regularly as a form of slowing down the spread of the COVID-19 is one of the recommended prophylactic measures by the WHO. However, some of the population in Nigeria, for instance, believe that using hot water to wash your hands will get germs off better than cold water. This myth, not supported by evidence, was an obstacle to implement the proven practice to simply wash hands with soap and running water for a long enough time (minimum of 20 s) and to dry your hands afterward.

Evolution of COVID-19

The United Nations Economic Commission for Africa in April 2020 expressed the fear that even with social distancing, the continent of Africa could have nearly 123 million cases of COVID-19 in 2020 and that 300,000 people may die of the disease. They went further to state that many health systems in Africa are ill equipped. Challenges include inconsistent power supply with the dependency of some hospitals on generators, shortages of essential workers, such as anesthetists, intensivists, and critical care nurses much needed during the pandemic.[5] Similarly, Reuters reported the scarcity of critical care beds and ventilators, counting with one or less for every 100,000 people. Some countries such as Guinea-Bissau were reputed to have no ventilators at all.[6] In Uganda, there are only 55 functional intensive care unit (ICU) beds to serve the 40 million people (1.3 ICU beds per million population), 80% of which are located in the nation's capital city with an estimated nurse to patient ratio of 1:8.[7]

As of May 2020, there were more than 5 million confirmed cases of COVID-19 in the world surpassing 300,000 deaths. The United States of America, with a population of 330 million, contributed more than 30% of confirmed cases and deaths.[8] All 54 African countries have had reported cases of COVID-19 disease and the African continent with over 100,000 confirmed cases, 20% of them reported in South Africa (Johns Hopkins University's world map). The Johns Hopkins University further reported that other highly affected African countries were Egypt, Morocco, and Algeria.[9]

The WHO African Regional Office, on May 19, 2020, reported on its official Twitter handle @WHOAFRO that South Africa, Algeria, and Nigeria were countries with the highest COVID-19 prevalence in Africa. However, Lesotho had only one confirmed case with no deaths.[10] Nigeria, with a population of 200 million, on May 23, 2020, had 7520 confirmed cases with 221 fatalities. This was, however, increased to 27,564 confirmed cases with 616 deaths by July 4, 2020, while the global figure at the same time had risen to over 10 million and over half a million deceased. Meanwhile, the infection rate in the United States is even about 46 times greater than what is recorded so far in Africa. All these figures, could be deceivingly suggestive of Africa being "safer" than the rest of the world, something that requires deeper analysis.

There are also differences accounted among the different sub-Saharan countries. The index case of COVID-19 in Nigeria was reported on February 27, 2020 in Lagos, a 44-year-old traveler arrived at the Murtala Muhammed International Airport, at 10 P.M. Subsequently, several imported cases were detected at temperature screening points in International Airports and by cases of local population returning from trips who developed high-grade fever and sore throat. Surveillance was then heightened at the points of entry, and the list of high-risk countries was revised. Since March 17, 2020, the clusters of cases initially linked to travelers that had recently returned from the United Kingdom, the United States, France, and Spain evolved into community transmission of COVID-19.

In May 2020, Nigeria conducted about 38,000 tests, while Ghana conducted more than 184,000 tests. Both countries reported approximately 7000 positive results. Meanwhile, as Nigeria reported by that time 200 deaths, Ghana posted about 30 deceased.[9]

In other parts of the continent, in countries like Kenya, as stated by the United Nations Development Program, COVID-19 represents more than a health crisis, as the pandemic impact in the economy, politics, and social life will leave behind deep scars.[11] Kenya reported its first COVID-19 case on March 13, 2020, and by March 31, 2020, the number of confirmed cases has risen to 59, with over 70% of infections in Nairobi. As at April 22, 2020, the number of confirmed cases has increased to 303, nearly fivefold jump in the case count, i.e., the highest number of positive cases among the East African Community (EAC) member states. In the EAC countries, (Kenya, Uganda, Tanzania, Rwanda, and South Sudan) with a consistent and transparent reporting system, the numbers are only expected to rise as the governments roll out mass testing.[12]

Epidemiology and surveillance

Since February 27, 2020, the outbreak of COVID-19 in Lagos State, Nigeria, has spread geographically as the numbers relentlessly increased. The evolution of the outbreak shows that the trend has not followed the projected paths of an outbreak with doubling time of seven days. However, the interventions implemented, including the "lockdown" has slowed the rise in the number of cases. However, the average reproductive number remains two (one confirmed case infects at least two other people).

In Nigeria, the majority of the infected people are males (60%). In both genders, the most of the infected cases are from the age group 31–40 years. The average age is 36 years old with the minimum age of 6 weeks and maximum age of 78 years old.[13]

There is also a great variation in the number of fatalities but significantly lower reports compared to countries such as the United States, Italy, or Spain. As of May 23, 2020, the percentage of fatality in Nigeria was 0.0000012%, while the percentage of fatality in the United States was 0.00029%.[8] A factor that could have contributed to these differences might be the average age of the infected population, younger in Nigeria compared to the United States and Western Europe. In addition to these, the presence of comorbidities in the latter countries compared to the predominant positive reports in Africa.

Political governance and COVID-19

Most African governments rose up to fight against the scourge of the COVID-19 infectivity as soon as it was declared a pandemic by the WHO, by restricting international travel even before a case was reported in their nations.[14] Lagos State is the epicenter of the COVID-19 pandemic in Nigeria, where the Federal Government supported the efforts of the Lagos State authorities by giving them a financial aid of N10 Billion of Nigerian Dollars (equivalent to approximately 2.4 million US dollars) to help contain the COVID-19 pandemic.

One of the strategies employed by many African countries includes the construction of isolation centers in various capital cities and areas of high prevalence of the disease. The central governments, through the Presidential Task Force on COVID-19, in Nigeria or the Ghana's Emergency Preparedness and Response Project, assist various committees in prevention, surveillance, and treatment protocols for the containment of the COVID-19 pandemic in the various African countries.

The United States and Western Europe introduced the policy of "lockdown" as a strategy to lower the incidence of fatalities and containment of the viral scourge. In a similar fashion, many African countries, including Nigeria, introduced the same policy of "lockdown" when it was evident that the number of infected cases was increasing.

Furthermore, as Africa faces the COVID-19 challenge, international agencies such as the African Development Bank, based in Côte d'Ivoire, have responded proactively to support African countries by approving a $10 billion crisis response facility to support African countries.[15] This is premised on the fact that many African countries, particularly those already dealing with high levels of debt, carry financial challenges, constraining their ability to respond to the COVID-19 crisis. In addition, this facility will assist in the provision of food relief and restoring the livelihoods of vulnerable populations severely affected by COVID-19. Also, this facility will complement ongoing activities of African governments to mitigate the effects of the virus pandemic on Africans.

The Joint United Nations Program on human immunodeficiency virus/acquired immunodeficiency syndrome was reported as saying that beating COVID-19 in Africa is the key to overcoming it globally. It went further to state that the greatest risk will be to poor people in resource-limited countries who are already battling other diseases such as human immunodeficiency virus/acquired immunodeficiency syndrome and tuberculosis.[16]

Advances in management of COVID-19

The COVID-19 disease has no cure presently, but the advanced countries like United States and countries in Western Europe had been trying all kinds of drug combinations to supportively manage the disease. In the early days of the pandemic, some of these drugs include the use of antiretroviral drugs such as *Kaletra* (lopinavir/ritonavir), zinc, chloroquine, and hydroxychloroquine. Recently, the WHO warned against the use of chloroquine to treat the COVID-19 disease.

One of the tropical countries in Africa, Madagascar, has blazed the trail by launching the global "herbal medicine" business by manufacturing their *Artemisia* extract, called "COVID-Organics", for the treatment of COVID-19 infection. They have exported this "wonder" herbal drug to various African and European countries, while the WHO itself has now shown interest in it.[17]

Also, during the lockdown, the Rwandan government has introduced robots in the fight against COVID-19 at some of its treatment centers as a way of decreasing contact between medical personnel and patients as a barrier to the transmission of the infection. The robots are expected to be involved in testing for coronavirus and in the distribution of medicines. They are also involved in the administration of the isolation centers. On May 19, 2020, Rwanda has reported 11 confirmed cases and 6 recoveries. So far, the country has conducted 52,335 tests by that time.[18]

According to the WHO, the lack of coronavirus tests is one of the biggest problems of the African continent. Senegal has developed a test kit with an estimated cost of less than USD10, and they are in the process of packaging it and distributing to African countries.[19] Ghana has developed drones for the quick retrieval and delivery of swab samples from the various test centers around the country.

Research and treatment prospects

Remdesivir, an antiviral drug, has been recommended for use in the United States and Europe for the treatment of COVID-19, making it the first drug to be approved for treatment.[20] It has been shown to reduce the time to discharge. It is recommended for its use in adults and adolescents from 12 years of age with pneumonia who require oxygen support. However, it may take significant time for this drug to be available in Africa because of its costs (over $5000 per course in the United States). It is available as an intravenous preparation, but there are plans of having the drug as an easier-to-use inhaled version.

Another drug that was recently introduced in the United Kingdom following a successful clinical trial by the "Oxford" Group, is the well-known steroid, dexamethasone, an antiinflammatory drug that acts as a modulator of inflammatory mediators.[21] It is cheap and widely available making it attractive to most countries especially after it has shown benefits when used in patients with moderate-to-severe COVID-19 disease who are on the ventilator or receiving oxygen therapy. This drug regimen has been validated by several study groups through clinical trials in the COVID-19 ICUs in Nigeria.

Challenges

With the increasing number of COVID-19-positive patients in most African countries, the bed availability in isolation centers is becoming inadequate. In Nigeria, the construction of these isolation and treatment centers is very expensive. This led the Federal Government of Nigeria, through the Nigeria Centre for Disease Control (NCDC) to devise a new protocol of discharging home COVID-19-positive patients after testing negative once in the course of their treatment in the isolation center. Furthermore, the Lagos State Emergency Operations Center, following the increasing numbers of positive patients and still being the epicenter of the pandemic in Nigeria, has brought out their policy of "home-based" care. This new protocol rolled out in the last week of June 2020, based on the fact that many COVID-19 patients, especially the asymptomatic ones or those with mild disease, they typically refuse admission to these isolation centers for various reasons. The new protocol thus ensures admission to the isolation centers is limited to only those with moderate-to-severe COVID-19 disease.

Stigmatization is another big challenge in the management of COVID-19-positive patients in Africa. This accounts for many people refusing testing, especially during the phase of active case search in the community. This is a reason for refusal of evacuation of COVID-19-positive patients to the isolation centers, especially with the arrival of an ambulance at their residence with health workers fully dressed in the personal protective equipment outfit. In Africa, the challenge of testing the population is not a minor detail. In Nigeria, like in most African countries, only the molecular biology testing technique using the confirmatory polymerase chain reaction test is approved to use. However, there is a recurrent shortage and sometimes lack of availability of sampling and extraction kits, which are generally supplied by the WHO, through the NCDC in Nigeria.

Another important challenge is the access to oxygen and critical care beds. Most of the COVID-19-positive and symptomatic patients end up with respiratory hypoxemia and will require oxygen therapy, but this is not universally available outside state capitals or big cities. This is largely because of the nondevelopment of health infrastructure in most African countries. However, from anecdotal reports, the number of COVID-19-positive patients that required ICU admission is very low compared to the numbers reported by the United States and Western Europe. Presently, following more knowledge about the pathophysiology of the COVID-19 in the lungs, emphasis is now on noninvasive positive pressure ventilation, making use of the mechanical ventilator a last resource in the management of severe cases of COVID-19.

The burden of noncommunicable diseases such as diabetes, hypertension, and traffic crash injuries has been relatively high and worrisome in most African countries, especially south of the Sahara. However, the advent of the COVID-19 pandemic has shifted spending on these diseases and impacted on the successes being recorded in this health sector.

The travel restrictions resulting from the COVID-19 pandemic is already affecting Africa's economy and developmental efforts. Most African countries depend on tourism to boost their revenue. Following this challenge, the economic growth in Africa has been predicted to decline by 2.1%–5.1% this year.[22] Business travel is also constrained, and if the business sector is weak, it will affect the aviation industry. The airlines have been grounded as a result of the lockdown imposed in most countries, and this also affected the intercity vehicular transportation. It will be difficult for African airlines to get the proverbial "bailouts" from governments after the pandemic is contained and the lockdowns eased. However, it is a well-known fact that Africa remains a destination for a lot of people around the world. Hopefully, the aviation industry in Africa will be rejuvenated once the pandemic is over.

Conclusions

The COVID-19 pandemic, caused by the novel coronavirus disease, is a big challenge and posed a major burden on the African continent. The projection of the Western world that the upsurge in confirmed COVID-19 cases would weaken the health systems, and even the political stability of African nations has, however, not been the case, so far. Several theories for this have been propagated, but the BCG vaccination policy of countries with low case and fatality rates seems to be the most favored in this regard, as validated by a multicountry level study.

There are various implications and challenges in the COVID-19 pandemic and its impact on Africa as well as in its containment. These include chiefly economic challenges and those linked to sociopolitical matters such as stigmatization of patients who tested positive to the virus and the state of the health infrastructure of the nations. Furthermore, COVID-19 has shifted focus from other noncommunicable killer diseases such as high blood pressure, diabetes, road traffic injuries that are the main killers in most African countries. It is hoped that health budgets of African countries may have to be reviewed in order to cater for the control of these noncommunicable diseases.

The pathophysiology and treatment options for the coronavirus disease are still evolving. With increased testing capacities, it remains to be seen whether the projected increase in number of COVID-19 patients will overtly overwhelm the health indices of African countries or not, in the face of global search for vaccines as well as the provision of support for the containment of the pandemic by international agencies like the African Development Bank.

References

1. Heininger U, Seward JF. Varicella. *Lancet.* 2006;368:1365–1376.
2. Lee BW. Review of varicellar zoster sero-epidemiology in India and Southeast Asia. *Trop Med Int Health.* 1998;3:886–890.
3. Cuccinotta D, Vanelli M. WHO declares COVID-19 a pandemic. *Acta Biomed.* 2020;91:157–160.
4. Katbi M, Adeoye O, Adedoyin A, et al. A multicountry level comparison of BCG vaccination policy and COVID-19 cases and mortality. *J Infect Dis Epidemiol.* 2020;6(3):131. https://doi.org/10.23937/2474-3658/1510131.
5. United Nations Economic Commission for Africa (UNECA). https://health.economictimes.indiatimes.com/news/industry/virus-exposes-gaping-holes-in-africas-health-systems/75599490. Accessed 25 May 2020.
6. Reuters Survey. https://www.reuters.com/news/picture/exclusive-virus-exposes-gaping-holes-in-idUSKBN22J1GZ.
7. Atumanya P, Sendagire C, Wabule A, et al. Assessment of the current capacity of intensive care units in Uganda: a descriptive study. *J Crit Care.* 2020;59:95–99.
8. COVID-19 Update. *Cable News Network (CNN)*; 2020.
9. Johns Hopkins University World Map. https://coronavirus.jhu.edu/map.html. Accessed 22 May 2020.
10. *Twitter @WHOAFRO*; 2020.
11. United Nations Development Program (UNDP). https://www.undp.org/content/undp/en/home/coronavirus.html.
12. Were M. *COVID-19 and Socio-Economic Impact in Africa-the Case of Kenya.* UNU-Wider; 2020. https://doi.org/10.35188/UNU-WIDER/WBN/2020-3.
13. *Corona Virus Disease (COVID-19) Outbreak Situation Report.* Lagos Emergency Operations Centre (EOC), Lagos State Ministry of Health; 2020. 5 May.
14. Macamo E. The Normality of Risk: African and European Responses to Covid-19. *Corona Times.* 2020. April 13 https://www.coronatimes.net/normality-risk-african-european-responses/. Accessed 23 May 2020.
15. *African Development Bank Group's Covid-19 Rapid Response Facility (CRF)*; 2020. Available at https://www.afdb.org/en/covid-19. Accessed 28 May 2020.

16. HEALTHTIMES; 2020. 19 May. Available at: https://healthtimes.co.zw/2020/05/19/op-ed-we-will-not-defeat-covid-19-without-including-africa-in-the-global-response/. Accessed 19 May 2020.
17. *WHO to Study Madagascar's Drug to Treat Covid-19.* Available at https://www.aa.com.tr/en/africa. Accessed 28 May 2020.
18. Johns Hopkins University World Map. https://coronavirus.jhu.edu/map.html. Accessed 19 May 2020.
19. *Senegal Develops COVID-19 Test Kits For Africa.* Available at www.healthwise.senegal.punchng.com. Accessed 29 May 2020.
20. *Gilead's Remdesivir Endorsed as First COVID-19 Treatment in Europe.* Medscape; 2020. 25 June.
21. *Dexamethasone Hailed as 'Breakthrough' in COVID-19 Trial, Reduced Deaths.* Medscape; 2020. 16 June.
22. Madden P. *Figures of the Week: The Macroeconomic Impact of COVID-19 in Africa;* 2020. Available at https://www.brookings.edu/blog/africa-in-focus/2020/04/16/figures-of-the-week-the-macroeconomic-impact-of-covid-19-in-africa/. Accessed 28 May 2020.

How the Middle East is facing COVID-19

19

Ahmed Reda Taha

Cleveland Clinic Lerner College of Medicine, Case Western Reserve University, Critical Care Institute, Cleveland Clinic Abu Dhabi, Abu Dhabi, United Arab Emirates

Introduction

Despite varying levels of health system infrastructure that reflect on preparedness across the region, Middle East and North Africa (MENA) countries' overall health management strategies, characterized by strict containment measures enforced early in the outbreak, efficiently controlled the pandemic's emerging spread in the region. As of June, countries are progressively and carefully getting down to ease restrictions on movement and economic activities and prepare their strategy toward deconfinement.

The MENA region's governmental authority has taken short aggressive measures to limit the spread of coronavirus disease 2019 (COVID-19) infection by limiting many innumerable individuals' movements. Their square measure over 800,000 confirmed cases across the MENA region, with a substantial proportion (30%) in Iran. Among Arab economies, the Kingdom of Saudi Arabia has the highest confirmed cases, followed by Qatar and the United Arab Emirates (UAE).[1]

COVID-19 is the second coronavirus that affects the Middle East, following the Middle East respiratory syndrome coronavirus reported in Saudi Arabia in 2012. UAE was the first Middle Eastern country to say a case, following the COVID-19 happening in China. The Middle East faces the dual threats of potential mass virus outbreaks in conflict zones and looming socioeconomic upheaval. Each crisis might have severe humanitarian consequences.

MENA region has reacted preemptively, and this contributed to flattening the curve of infections in their countries. Most of the Arab countries implementing social distancing measures while the virus was still in its infancy. Meanwhile, Saudi Arabia adopted an aggressive approach toward the virus, including a curfew from nightfall to dawn. National capital conjointly adopted alternative radical steps like preventing holy journey to two of Islam's most religious places—Mecca and Medina.[1]

COVID-19 Pandemic. https://doi.org/10.1016/B978-0-323-82860-4.00008-2

Outbreak and management of the health crisis

The increasing spread of the coronavirus across countries has prompted many governments to introduce unprecedented containment measures to reduce community impact. These are priority measures enforced by a sanitary situation, which leaves little room for other sectors as health should remain the primary concern.

The containment measures achieved with rapid identification and isolation of suspect or confirmed COVID-19 cases. Associated with strict infection control measures to minimize intrahospital transmission and prevent incapacitation of essential services, the planned response is a continuum and will vary based on the scale and severity of the pandemic.

The first COVID-19 cases in MENA countries observed in the UAE. According to numbers exaggerated sharply within the first few weeks of the happening, the worldwide trend is in line with numbers. However, infection and mortality rates could seem to the point that the pandemic has not hit the region as laborious. The number of COVID-19-related deaths in Arab countries, compared to the population, remains so much below the rates recorded in some European and Asian countries.[2]

These measures will be explained by MENA economies' swift and early response. Following the pandemic, they introduced strict containment measures beginning within the half of March. Notably, several countries did not wait to own confirmed cases to impose movement restrictions and social distancing measures. For example, Saudi Arabia suspended pilgrimages to Mecca and Medina and barred access to holy sites within the two cities as early as March.[2]

Most countries started closing colleges and nurseries and prohibiting giant public gatherings, together with spiritual ones. Given the pandemic risk, many countries declared a state of national emergency and obligatory stricter containment measures and necessary self-isolation and curfews. All countries have banned entry to foreigners till additional notice, and air traffic has been placed on hold or considerably reduced. Borders stay open for the transport of products and medical instrumentality. Quarantine rules are including severe penalties for noncompliance, starting from fines to jail sentencing, like in Jordan, Saudi Arabia, and the UAE.[2,3]

As of May, many MENA countries have begun to relax confinement measures bit by bit and set up their exit ways. Deconfinement plans were either progressive, like Lebanon's five-step reopening set up that started on April 27, or depend on a geographical breakdown between low-risk and speculative regions, because it is that the case in the Asian country that has been divided into white, yellow, and red areas based on the number of confirmed infections and deaths. Algeria, Bahrain, Iraq, Lebanon, Saudi Arabia, and also the UAE have all approved businesses and commercial places to resume activity, at least partly. These measures raise the cases in Kingdom of Saudi Arabia, and they change the plan to strict confinement.[3,4]

MENA region proposed a plan that leads to the success of its containment ways to approach the deconfinement part. The gradual easing of restrictions has been associated with permanent strict preventive measures. Physical distancing is enforced in most countries, with businesses comply with preventative measures. Face masks have conjointly been mandatory in public places in Bahrain, Morocco, Qatar, and also the UAE, with violators facing significant penalties, together with up to jail.[4]

Challenges to health systems and health sector responses

MENA countries' containment efforts have proved a diversity of responses in light of the region's varying levels of health system preparedness.

Over the past 25 years, the Gulf Cooperation Council (GCC) countries have undertaken substantial investments in health-care infrastructure, aboard efforts to extend the number of doctors and nursing personnel. This has considerably improved the standard of health-care services within the GCC. In an assessment of COVID-19 preparedness published in March by the World Health Organization (WHO), where countries were graded on a scale of one to five, with one that means no capacity to retort and five that means sustainable capacity, all GCC countries except Qatar scored either four or five. However, GCC health systems face many challenges as well as vital risk factors associated with lifestyle diseases like diabetes, obesity, and cardiovascular diseases. Especially, diabetes prevalence rates within the region are among the highest worldwide as high as 22% in Kuwait and 18.3% in Saudi Arabia. As diabetes and obesity are reported to be a risk factor for hospitalization and mortality of the COVID-19 infection, this could place an extra strain on GCC health systems' capacity to respond to the crisis. Another concern is GCC's significant reliance on expatriate medical hands and foreign medical equipment and supplies, which can be affected by travel and transport restrictions.[4]

Developing MENA economies have suffered from insufficient health resources, shortages of skilled faculty within the health-care system, and lack of enough medical equipment. Total health expenditure per capita in the majority of MENA countries is considerably below average for countries in similar financial gain categories. Moreover, the quantity of physicians per 1000 inhabitants within the region is substantially below the WHO suggested threshold of 4.5 doctors, nurses, and midwives per 1000 population and as low as 0.72 and 0.79 in Morocco and Egypt, respectively.[4]

For countries suffering to maintain basic life requirements and political conflict, the COVID-19 pandemic poses exceptionally fragile and uncoordinated responses in these areas. It lacks the mandatory capability to react to the crisis in terms of medical facilities, equipment, and personnel. In Syria, the WHO estimates that 70% of health-care workers have left the country as migrants or refugees. In comparison, only 64% of hospitals and 52% of primary health-care centers remain fully operational.[1]

MENA governments introduced measures and dedicated specific funds to stop their health systems from being overwhelmed and cut back the fast spread of COVID-19, to support their medical staff and protect the community. Many countries have enhanced the number of critical care units and hospital beds to admit COVID-19 patients, as well as by building dedicated treatment facilities as within

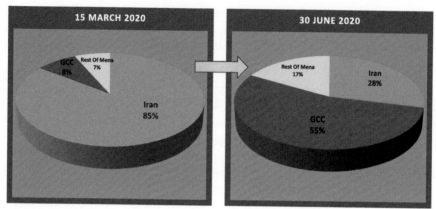

FIG. 1

Comparing the progress of COVID-19 patient's distribution across the MENA region from March to June 2020.[6,7]

the UAE, that performs quite 40,000 tests/day. Governments have conjointly scaled up their testing capability by creating new sites and establishing drive-through testing stations. This has enabled countries to facilitate detection, tracing, and isolation of cases[5] (Fig. 1).

Statistics across the region

As of June 28, 2020, the total number of COVID-19 cases in MENA region reached 800,000. With 235,000 confirmed COVID-19 cases, Iran is the regional epicenter of the new coronavirus, and the country's case numbers have grown exponentially since March 25, when it had about 24,811 cases. However, as the coronavirus has spread across the region, Iran's share in the total number of MENA cases has reduced from 86% on March 25 to 30% as of June 28 with a total death cases of 11,408. Middle Eastern governments, led by the GCC, are conducting more intensive health screening operations to identify potential cases of the illness. To date, Saudi Arabia, the second in COVID-19 cases with the total number currently 206,000, has recorded 143,000 recoveries and 1885 deaths related to COVID-19.[6,7]

The third in the region is Qatar with 99,000 cases followed by Egypt 72,000 cases, it is the worst-hit country in terms of case numbers outside Iran and the GCC.

While health experts have warned that the easing of restrictions could cause a second wave of COVID-19 in the country, most of the countries' government says it must resume activity to buoy its sanction-hit economy (Fig. 2).

To date, 610,00 individuals in the MENA region have recovered from COVID-19 with 76% of the total cases, while 19,400 individuals have died of the illness.[6,7]

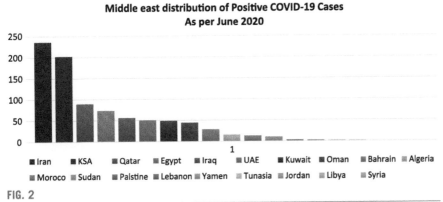

FIG. 2

The COVID-19 patients' distribution across the MENA region as of June 2020.[6,7]

Governments' strategic responses

Following the confirmation of the first cases of COVID-19 within the MENA region, national governments quickly adopted measures to strengthen institutional coordination by making interministerial structures.

Other measures include the creation of technical and scientific committees in charge of monitoring and evaluating the progress of the situation and anticipating the direct and indirect repercussions of COVID-19. For example, the Tunisian government has created a National COVID-19 Monitoring Authority, gathering senior officials from all ministries, with the aim of "imposing full compliance with measures to fight the virus." The authority will also ensure the coordination between the National Committee against the coronavirus, headed by the Presidency of the Government, and the regional committees against natural catastrophes. It will also be in charge of "monitoring the regularity of the supply of basic products, the distribution of social assistance to poor families or families without income, as well as the referral of recommendations to the national committee to combat COVID-19 to adopt the necessary measures to contain the virus".[8]

Many governments also adopted measures to ensure the continuity of public services in countries where confinement measures were imposed. Teleworking arrangements and online tools have been developed to facilitate the ongoing functioning of public administration. Jordan and Morocco developed practical manuals on teleworking, outlining crucial advice and tips to facilitate its use. Morocco also created a series of new digital delivery services that aim to reduce the exchange of paper documents, thus limiting the risk of COVID-19 transmission via papers.[8]

In the Gulf region, the authority enhances teleworking for most of the government sectors and provides an online portal to strengthen the confinement.

Multiple categories rapidly took place on a large scale for the pandemic, including infection control; intensive care unit (ICU) bed surge capacity; adequate staffing of physicians, nurses, and respiratory therapists; complicated ethical dilemmas; and staff wellness. Procedures to deal with these problems were created and enforced together with nursing, respiratory therapist, and hospital leadership.[9]

Patient characteristics

Age is a strong risk factor for severity, complications, and death. Patients in the Middle East with no reported underlying medical conditions had an overall case fatality of 0.9% similar to international figure. Patients with comorbidities encounter higher case fatalities: those with cardiovascular disease, those with diabetes, and chronic respiratory disease, or cancer, prior stroke, chronic lung disease, and chronic kidney disease have all been associated with increased severity and adverse outcomes. Serious heart conditions, including heart failure, coronary artery disease, congenital heart disease, cardiomyopathies, and pulmonary hypertension, may put people at higher risk for severe illness from COVID-19. People with hypertension may be at an increased risk for severe illness from COVID-19 and should continue to take their medications as prescribed. At this time, people who have only underlying medical condition like hypertension are not considered to be at higher risk for severe illness from COVID-19.[10]

Accounting for differences in age, prevalence of the underlying condition, and mortality associated with COVID-19 reported in the Middle East country till now has been similar to reports from the United States and China.

The typical course of the disease

Most patients admitted to the ICU have similar presentations with fever, difficult breathing, and cough as a classic triad that can be associated with other nonspecific symptoms of generalized malaise, myalgia, and diarrhea.[11]

Typically, patients started to be symptomatic after day 5 with the progressive difficulty of breathing and desaturation to <90% (detected by pulse oximeter), and in day 10, high requirement of oxygen using high-flow nasal cannula, BiPAP, is the next feature for most of the patients. Response to different therapy and self-proning has different effects but usually show initial response. By the end of 2 weeks, most of the patients who didn't improve become intubated with a classic presentation of acute respiratory distress syndrome (ARDS).

Lung compliance earlier may not be compromised but within 1 week of intubation mostly dropped to less than 20. Multiple studies are currently running to support these data[11] (Fig. 3).

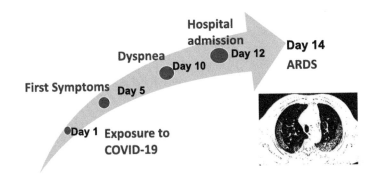

FIG. 3

The trend of COVID-19 presentation as recorded across the MENA region.

Clinical challenges

Currently, there are no drugs or other therapeutics approved by the U.S. Food and Drug Administration or recommended by WHO to prevent or treat COVID-19. Current clinical management includes infection prevention and control measures and supportive care, including supplemental oxygen and mechanical ventilatory support when indicated and most of the available drugs included under investigational clinical trial.

Multiple clinical challenges arise with the pandemic everywhere across the Middle East countries, and it dictates special precautions to maximize patient outcomes and minimize the chance to spread the disease to intensive care practitioners.

A comprehensive airway management policy was adapted from rapidly evolving international recommendations.[12,13] These procedures ensured that the most experienced staff would attempt intubation using a video laryngoscope and rapid sequence induction (RSI). To improve efficiency and optimize patient care, a critical care physician, when identified a patient who required intubation, that physician notified the COVID-19 intubation team. Preparations included obtaining induction, sedation, and vasopressor medications; ensuring the use of appropriate personal protective equipment (PPE) for this high-risk procedure (impervious gown, goggles, or welder's mask, gloves, head covers, and papers); the team moving the patient to a negative-pressure room for intubation. The initial team included an anesthesiologist, a critical care nurse, and a respiratory therapist. Patients as per recommendations should be intubated using RSI and a video laryngoscope. The multidisciplinary critical care team then moved the patient to the intensive care unit (ICU).

Additional methods evolved due to an increased number of hospital admissions and intubations, by involving two anesthesia airway groups covering 24h a day, 7days a week, dedicated to COVID-19 intubations. This team brought with them the acceptable PPE and a video-assisted intubation device. Hospital pharmacologists created virtual RSI kits to be easily accessed on each floor. Finally, a peri-intubation team led by certified registered nurse anesthetists assumed the role of coordinative peri-intubation procedures, as well as gathering medications and staff and transporting patients to the negative-pressure room before intubation and also to the ICU after intubation.

Role of infectious disease consultants

Given the highly infectious nature of the disaster and the rapidly evolving therapeutic landscape, infectious disease consultants instantly established a dedicated COVID-19 team. This team consults on every critically sick patient with COVID-19 daily to review infectious disease parameters and advice regarding therapies (antiviral and antimicrobial)[14] and trying detection of patients susceptible to cytokine storming syndrome and propose innovative therapies.[15,16] Moreover, they show evolving therapeutic trials[17] (Table 1).

Extracorporeal organ support

Institutional policies concerning extracorporeal membrane oxygenation (EMCO) are evolving with the publication of efficacy and risk information.[18] Although EMCO has shown potential benefit in a subset of patients with COVID-19, the choice to cannulate must include the ability to provide appropriate staffing and resources. Potential candidates are discussed on a case-by-case basis in a multidisciplinary fashion. The renal replacement has been offered to all or any patients with acute or chronic renal failure via conventional hemodialysis, continuous renal replacement therapy, or peritoneal dialysis, with associate awareness of the resources concerned in every situation.[19]

Cardiac arrests

Given the virulent nature of the novel coronavirus, approaches to resuscitation have evolved.[19,20] As such, institutional cardiopulmonary resuscitation policies were instituted that restricted the number of responders to cardiac arrests outside the ICU. Mechanical compression devices were rapidly introduced to cut back further the number of staff responding to the code. Furthermore, the responding team should carry a COVID-19 pack to every cardiac arrest, which included high-risk PPE (face shields, N95 masks, PAPR, and impermeable gowns) considering the aerosolizing nature of cardiopulmonary resuscitation. Resuscitations within the ICU still are conducted in an exceedingly standard fashion, with attempts to minimize aerosolization by leaving the patient on the ventilator or, if necessary, using a bag valve mask with a high-efficiency particulate air filter attached to the expiratory port.[20]

Table 1 Recommended infection prevention general measures.

General measures
- Develop robust risk stratification criteria
- Actively identify and isolate patients suspected to have COVID-19
- Effective contact tracing
- Rapid laboratory diagnostic testing
- Care for suspected or confirmed cases in negative pressure AIIR—patients to wear face masks until transfer to AIIRs
- Strict hand hygiene and standard precautions
- Staff PPE requirements
- For all patients: droplet and standard precautions, with additional airborne precautions when performing aerosol-generating procedures
- For suspected/known COVID-19 patients: droplet, contact, and airborne precautions
- Fit testing for all staff using N95 respirators
- Staff training (and retraining) for appropriate use, donning, and removal of PPE, with pictorial guides and videos where applicable
- Stockpile PPE and consumables for infection control
- Single-use items for patients (e.g., disposable blood pressure cuff)
- Disinfect shared equipment after use
- Provision of (disposable) staff scrub suits in isolation wards
- Appropriate handling of medical waste
- Hospital issued guidelines for infection prevention, including handling of patient specimens and care of the deceased patient
- Staff segregation and physical distancing
- Centrally tracked staff surveillance (e.g., temperature monitoring) and access to designated staff clinics
- Reduce face-to-face encounters with patients (e.g., video monitoring, telemedicine, wearables for vital sign monitoring)
- Minimize patient movement or transport
- Exclude visitors to patients with suspected or known COVID-19
- Restrict unnecessary attendance at hospitals (e.g., medical students, members of public, research coordinators)
- Minimize or postpone elective admissions and operations
- *Droplet and Contact PPE:*
- *Surgical mask, eye protection, disposable gown, gloves, and cap*
- *Droplet, Contact and Airborne PPE:*
- *N95 respirator (consider PAPR use), eye protection, disposable gown, gloves, and cap*

Abbreviations: COVID-19, coronavirus disease 2019; AIIR, airborne infection isolation room; PPE, personal protective equipment; PAPR, powered air-purifying respirator; NIV, noninvasive ventilation; HFNC, high-flow nasal cannula therapy; ICU, intensive care unit.[17]

Standardization of care across critical supply areas

Given the speedy growth of the ICU and the sizable number of caregivers concerned within the management of critically ill patients with COVID-19, frequent formal and informal communication among all the teams has been essential. This communication is especially necessary as a result of having clinicians from other driplines who do not routinely care for patients with ARDS. Daily evaluation and assessment by one of the critical care team to all of the assigned areas outside the medical ICU become mandatory to optimize care for these patients. The development and distribution of informal guidelines outlining the fundamental aspects of caring for critically ill patients with COVID-19 have established to be valuable tools for providing standardized care in all areas. Secure electronic medical record file sharing and daily e-mail updates offer critical care providers easy accessibility to the newest hospital policies, statistics protocols, and guidelines.

Most of centers provide a lot of innovative ideas to save the intensivist time to help the most significant number of patients and keep the safety of the staff.[21,22]

Approaches to economic use of your time within the ICU

Dedicated mobile phone placed in every negative pressure room so that staff members within the area can contact extra staff outside the area while not doffing their PPE.

A dedicated procedure team comprised of anesthesiologists, surgeons, and interventional radiologists was created to perform ICU procedures like central line, arterial line, or nasogastric tube insertion around the clock. This helps the intensivists to facilitate acute patient care. A multidisciplinary tracheostomy procedure team led by thoracic surgery, otorhinolaryngology, and critical care specialists offer an equally centered approach to a different crucial essential aspect of care. A dedicated proning team was formed by clinical nurse specialists in critical care medicine and physical therapy to minimize the unit-specific staff needed for pronation or supination of patients while providing a standardized approach to this therapeutic maneuver.[23] In an innovative adaptation, current drips, ventilator settings, a summary of the daily plan, target ECMO parameters, and arterial blood gas results were written on the glass doors of the room so that staff could be informed without having to enter the room and relieving staff can easily share the plans. This technique was made possible by the restriction of visitors to the hospital.

Minimizing exposure to workers

Care has been bundled the maximum amount as possible. Laboratory sampling was regular with medication dosing. Larger baggage of intravenous fluid or additional focused solutions was used to limit the number of times a nurse had to enter the area. Imaging studies and ECGs were restricted to those deemed necessary. In some (but not all) rooms, intravenous pumps were placed outside the room with the utilization of additional intravenous tubing. Though this approach permits medications to be managed outside the room, its limitations embody the length of your time needed for a bolus to reach the patient. A buddy system including one staff member by the medication pumps became necessary to allow delivery of boluses or adjustments of medication to be made from outside the room while staff inside the room turned or cleaned the patient. The monitor for the most frequently used ventilators was detached and similarly kept outside the room. The advantages and drawbacks of these regulations are currently under study to evaluate how much it is effective.[24,25]

The health authorities in most of the MENA region ask physician and health-care providers to work remotely, employer's priority should be given to pregnant women, those aged 55 and above, those with disabilities, respiratory or chronic diseases and female workers who are mothers of children in grade 9 and below. Employers are also required to comply with the temporary guide for remote working in private sectors, which requires, for example, that the employer provides the relevant technical equipment to facilitate home working and determining mechanisms for the management of remote working. And staff who received anti-immunosuppression drugs to clearly identified themselves to be out of the COVID-19–treating areas.[25]

Education

Led by critical care physicians, started with techniques of donning and doffing properly to protect staff and nurse's patient safety and minimize cross-infection, a rapid simulation-based curriculum focused on pronation and COVID-19, managing aerosolized procedure, cardiac arrests was instituted and provided for both day- and night-shift nurses in nonmedical ICUs. Our provider teams have been monitoring the rapidly evolving diagnostic and therapeutic approaches in the global arena to improve and optimize care on a local level. Web-based conferences, referencing seminal articles on ARDS still be conducted often. Topics have enclosed ventilator management, fluid management, pronation for intubated and non-intubated patients, sedation, and paralysis, among others. Recommendations from international colleagues are discussed in these multidisciplinary conferences.

Exclusive teaching webinars arranged by most of the hospital to teach non – ICU physicians how to help in this pandemic and to achieve the maximum benefit of diploid physicians and nurses during their presence in the critical care unit.[26]

Efficient bed management

Bed assignments and unit-to-unit transfers are typically managed by a group of nurses and case managers in the operation center. This group is working in collaboration with our transfer center, which organizes the incoming transfer of patients from other hospitals. During this time of rapid expansion, one of the critical care physicians partnered with these nurses around the clock, on a rotating basis, to triage all critically ill patients to streamline bed assignments and facilitate transfers into the newly created ICUs.[27]

This outline provides an understanding of how critical care, in collaboration with and appreciation of other colleagues in the departments and divisions of pulmonary and critical care, anesthesiology, cardiology, neurocritical care, surgical critical care, hospital medicine, infectious diseases, palliative care, ethics, nursing, physical therapy, and respiratory therapy, are meeting this challenge. We provide potential guidelines for other centers to adapt as needed to help further streamline this expansion. The diploid physician from different department works in harmony with the critical care team to keep an adequate level of care.[27]

Communicating with families

The infectious nature of the COVID-19 pandemic has markedly impacted physicians' and staff's ability to speak with patients' families, an essential aspect of critical care. With limitations in visiting time, family communication has become complex and fragmented. To deal with this issue of patient care, a restricted number of patient relatives are designated to communicate with physicians. Besides, each family member is offered a second supportive call from a critical care team member. The critical care team discusses cases with each COVID-19 unit daily to assess for participating surrogates. In the setting of imminent death or immediately after death, a single family member in PPE is provided an opportunity to visit. If visitation is impossible, the staff can creatively use video conferencing to allow loved ones to visualize and speak to their dying family member.

Public relations departments and social workers should be involved to facilitate communication with family members or the public media, to minimize misunderstanding and build trust and confidence in the health-care system.[28]

While creating ICU surge capacity, the early patients with COVID-19 were admitted to negative-pressure rooms in the ICUs and divided among all of the ICUs. Initial surge plans were designed to accommodate an increased number of patients in the early stages, and later plans incorporated up to threefold higher numbers. For efficiency, we designated half of the beds as COVID-19 units. This call allowed units to adjust to COVID-19 patients before the complete unit was filled, allowed staff members to perfect donning and doffing techniques, provided a chance to position pumps and ventilator monitors outside the area, and enabled multiple staff members to develop experience in managing COVID-19.[29]

Maintaining ICU surge capacity

The current response will depend on available resources and trigger targets for activation of each phase of response should be defined early. At the end of the surge continuum, "emergency mass critical care practices" will have to be instituted, which may come at the cost of suboptimal standards of care. To mitigate acute ventilation shortage, we may use a high-flow nasal cannula therapy or noninvasive ventilation if we are facing acute ventilator shortages, even though they do not constitute evidence-based management due to infection control concerns (aerosolization of respiratory droplets). The triage of critically ill patients may become necessary to prioritize ICU resources and carefully consider ethical principles to ensure just and equitable delivery of care for all patients. Triaging protocols should not disadvantage patients without COVID-19 who need ICU care. Health-care systems must find a balance between "saving the most lives" and prioritizing care based on the probability of achieving clinical benefit. These criteria should ideally be objective, transparent, and publicly disclosed. Authorities should engage the community in this process so that public trust exists when it is most needed.[30,31]

Psychological burdens

This difficult pandemic has created tremendous ethical distress among critical care personnel. We tend to pride ourselves on the customized care of our patients. A challenging aspect of care during this pandemic was more than expected, giving the fact that the health-care provider does not really understand the nature of the disease, add to this unpredicted patient's loss, and many patients deteriorate fast in reverse to our expectation. The inability to produce care within the usual manner ordinarily involves patients' families as their network throughout their health problem. Critical care providers have expedited emotional life-altering conversations over video chats with relations and have watched families say goodbye without the advantage of privacy; the workers cannot leave the room without holding the phone or tablet. Physicians and nurses were minimizing their personal exposure to keep the balance being present and offering comfort for their patients. In addition to this heartbreaking reality, many providers work while watching this pandemic around us. Staffs fear for their health and that of their families. Many providers have isolated themselves either by staying in hotels or the hospital or by sending their family members away. Some have already created a will and advance directives for all of these psychological pressures and because of sheer exhaustion, recognizing that staff becomes overwhelmed with emotions ranging from anxiety to helplessness. To address these challenges, it has been vital to engage mental health-care providers with expertise in managing psychological trauma and acute stress as well as offering group and individual sessions to our staffs. Access to this service has been made as needed for psychological support, and staff members have been given an appointment with psychiatric professionals if required.[32]

Conclusions

Current situation showing a different distribution of severity as some of the Middle East countries achieved the flattening of the curve and others still in upsloping. It is challenging to evaluate the Middle East performance during COVID-19 pandemic while the process is still running. We can just enumerate the lessons learned from the start of this year till now.

Self-protection and personal hygiene measures need to be the overall attitude and principles for all the areas, which will require more investment in education and training. Avoiding overcrowding is mandatory and helps to flatten the curve and to contain the pandemic. Hospital admission should be only for symptomatic patients to save resources. No therapeutic options proved to be effective till now, so more research is required. Teamwork and effective communication are the influential factors that support the organizations in fighting against the pandemic.

Attention through all nations to the vital role of health-care providers and their requirement from training, upskilling, and that the current staff can meet the future need, and all of them operate in the highest level of their clinical competence.

Practical planning recommendations for specific interventions that communities may use for a given level of pandemic severity in case of the second surge, and the interim plan should suggest when and how these measures should be applied to minimize its overall burden to save people's life and prevent further economic crisis.

References

1. Tackling the coronavirus (COVID-19) crisis together: OECD policy contributions for co-ordinated action. *June 10. Retrieved July 6, 2020, from*; 2020. http://www.oecd.org/coronavirus/en/.
2. Salem P, Toukan DM. *March 23. MENA coronavirus update: The region faces an unprecedented crisis*; 2020. Retrieved July 06, 2020, from https://www.mei.edu/blog/mena-coronavirus-update-region-faces-unprecedented-crisis.
3. Azour J. *May 13. COVID-19 Pandemic and the Middle East and Central Asia: Region Facing Dual Shock*; 2020. Retrieved July 06, 2020, from https://blogs.imf.org/2020/03/23/covid-19-pandemic-and-the-middle-east-and-central-asia-region-facing-dual-shock/.
4. The National. *April 20. Coronavirus in the Middle East: Lockdowns extended across the region*; 2020. Retrieved July 06, 2020, from https://www.thenational.ae/world/mena/coronavirus-in-the-middle-east-lockdowns-extended-across-the-region-1.995673.
5. Wam. *June 24. Combating coronavirus: Mubadala's medical facilities in Abu Dhabi are now free of Covid-19 cases*; 2020. Retrieved July 06, 2020, from https://www.khaleejtimes.com/coronavirus-pandemic/combating-coronavirus-mubadalas-medical-facilities-in-abu-dhabi-are-now-free-of-covid-19-case.
6. Meeddubai. *April 06. Covid-19 cases top 465,000 in Mena*; 2020. Retrieved July 06, 2020, from https://www.meed.com/covid-19-cases-top-465000-in-mena.
7. Coronavirus Cases. *July 6. Retrieved July 06, 2020, from*; 2020. https://www.worldometers.info/coronavirus/?referer=app.
8. Policy Responses to COVID19. *July 2. Retrieved July 06, 2020, from*; 2020. https://www.imf.org/en/Topics/imf-and-covid19/Policy-Responses-to-COVID-19.
9. Griffin KM, Karas MG, Ivascu NS, Lief L. Hospital preparedness for COVID-19: a practical guide from a critical care perspective. *Am J Respir Crit Care Med.* 2020;201 (11):1337–1344. https://doi.org/10.1164/rccm.202004-1037cp.
10. Richardson S, Hirsch JS, Narasimhan M, et al. Presenting characteristics, comorbidities, and outcomes among 5700 patients hospitalized with COVID-19 in the new York City area. *JAMA.* 2020;323(20):2052. https://doi.org/10.1001/jama.2020.6775.

11. Chang D, Mo G, Yuan X, et al. Time kinetics of viral clearance and resolution of symptoms in novel coronavirus infection. *Am J Respir Crit Care Med.* 2020;201(9):1150–1152. https://doi.org/10.1164/rccm.202003-0524le.
12. Cook TM, El-Boghdadly K, McGuire B, McNarry AF, Patel A, Higgs A. *Consensus guidelines for managing the airway in patients with COVID-19: guidelines from the Difficult Airway Society, the Association of Anaesthetists the Intensive Care Society, the Faculty of Intensive Care Medicine and the Royal College of Anaesthetists. Anaesthesia [online ahead of print] 27 Mar*; 2020. https://doi.org/10.1111/anae.15054.
13. Orser BA. Recommendations for endotracheal intubation of COVID-19 patients. *Anesth Analg.* 2020;130:1109–1110.
14. Li H, Zhou Y, Zhang M, Wang H, Zhao Q, Liu J. Updated approaches against SARS-CoV-2. *Antimicrob Agents Chemother.* 2020. pii: AAC.00483–20.
15. Shen C, Wang Z, Zhao F, et al. Treatment of 5 critically ill patients with COVID-19 with convalescent plasma. *JAMA.* 2020. https://doi.org/10.1001/jama.2020.4783. [online ahead of print] 27 Mar.
16. Zhang B, Liu S, Tan T, et al. Treatment with convalescent plasma for critically ill patients with SARS-CoV-2 infection. *Chest.* 2020. pii: S0012–3692(20)30571–7.
17. Niederman MS, Richeldi L, Chotirmall SH, Bai C. Rising to the challenge of the novel COVID-19: advice for pulmonary and critical care and an agenda for research. *Am J Respir Crit Care Med.* 2020;201:1019–1022.
18. MacLaren G, Fisher D, Brodie D. Preparing for the most critically ill patients with COVID-19: the potential role of extracorporeal membrane oxygenation. *JAMA.* 2020;323:1245–1246.
19. Savary D, Morin F, Fadel M, Metton P, Richard JF, Descatha A. Considering the challenge of the Covid-19 pandemic, is there a need to adapt the guidelines for basic life support resuscitation? *Resuscitation.* 2020. pii: S0300–9572(20)30121–0.
20. Mahase E, Kmietowicz Z. Covid-19: doctors are told not to perform CPR on patients in cardiac arrest. *BMJ.* 2020;368:m1282.
21. Emanuel EJ, Persad G, Upshur R, et al. Fair allocation of scarce medical resources in the time of Covid-19. *N Engl J Med.* 2020. https://doi.org/10.1056/NEJMsb2005114. [online ahead of print] 23 Mar.
22. Gostin LO, Friedman EA, Wetter SA. Responding to COVID-19: how to navigate a public health emergency legally and ethically. *Hast Cent Rep.* 2020;50:8–12.
23. Pan C, Chen L, Lu C, et al. Lung recruitability in SARS-CoV-2 associated acute respiratory distress syndrome: a single-center, observational study. *Am J Respir Crit Care Med.* 2020. https://doi.org/10.1164/rccm.202003-0527LE. [online ahead of print] 23 Mar.
24. Diamond F. *March 09. Nurses | Infection Control Today*; 2020. Retrieved July 6, 2020, from https://www.infectioncontroltoday.com/nurses.
25. Khoja S. *June 28. Insight & Knowledge*; 2020. Retrieved July 06, 2020, from https://www.clydeco.com/insight/article/covid-19-middle-east-employment-an-update-on-new-government-initiatives.
26. Wallace D, Gillett B, Wright B, Stetz J, Arquilla B. Randomized controlled trial of high fidelity patient simulators compared to actor patients in a pandemic influenza drill scenario. *Resuscitation.* 2010;81:872–876.
27. Devereaux AV, Tosh PK, Hick JL, et al. Engagement and education: care of the critically ill and injured during pandemics and disasters: CHEST consensus statement. *Chest.* 2014;146:e118S–e133S.

28. Table of Contents - WHO. *Retrieved July 6, 2020, from*; 2017. https://www.who.int/mediacentre/communication-framework.pdf?ua=1.
29. Goh KJ, Wong J, Tien JC, et al. Preparing your intensive care unit for the COVID-19 pandemic: Practical considerations and strategies. *Crit Care*. 2020;24(1). https://doi.org/10.1186/s13054-020-02916-4.
30. Thompson AK, Faith K, Gibson JL, Upshur REG. Pandemic influenza preparedness: an ethical framework to guide decision-making. *BMC Med Ethics*. 2006;7:12.
31. Biddison LD, Berkowitz KA, Courtney B, et al. Ethical considerations: care of the critically ill and injured during pandemics and disasters: CHEST consensus statement. *Chest*. 2014;146:e145S–e155S.
32. Zawahir A. *May 08. Mental Health Burden During COVID-19: Anxiety, Depression, and Poor Sleep Quality*; 2020. Retrieved July 06, 2020, from https://www.psychiatryadvisor.com/home/topics/general-psychiatry/mental-health-burden-during-covid19-pandemic/.

COVID-19 pandemic in India

20

Kapil Zirpe and Sushma Gurav

Ruby Hall Clinic, Pune, Maharastra, India

India, officially the Republic of India is a country in South Asia. It is the second-most populous country, the seventh-largest country by land area, and the most populous democracy in the world.

Presently, India is ranking fourth in total coronavirus disease 2019 (COVID-19) patients so far detected in the world. Present mortality rate for India is around 3%.[1] We have trillion minds to tackle problem, but in case of COVID-19 pandemic where all developed countries had given up, we needed a tailor-made approach by keeping in mind our issues about the infrastructure in India (see Table 1). The tragedy is immediate, real, epic, and unfolding before our eyes. The COVID-19 tragedy is described as the wreckage of a train that has been careening down the track for years. European countries were already burning in this pandemic. To add to this, public health expenditure in India is just above 1% of gross domestic product (GDP) (4.8% of GDP if private health sector is considered).[2,3]

The warning signs of pandemic arrival in India were knocking our health-care system since the first few cases surfaced in Kerala (January 30, 2020).[4] All cases in Kerala had a history of travel to Wuhan. Screening at all airports of all the international passengers started on March 6. Indian Council of Medical Research didn't *t*-test people with COVID-19 symptoms without a recent travel history and a known contact that might have transmitted them the virus, up until March 20. The government's official line for the public as late as March 13 was that the coronavirus was not a health emergency.

Early signs of community spread were seen on March 10, 2020. On March 13 and 14, sequence of Covid-19-related events in India depicted in Table 2. India banned the entry of international travelers, visas were suspended for travel to India. All international travelers entering India were asked to self-quarantine for 14 days. India was one of the first countries to ban flights and ban travelers from China. Till March 15, 2020, Reverse transcription polymerase chain reaction tests were limited only to those who are symptomatic and those who gave abroad traveling history. Social distancing as a method of keeping the virus at bay was first officially flagged by the Prime Minister Narendra Modi when he spoke to the nation on March 19 in order to call for a 1-day "Janata Curfew" on March 22. The first national containment measure in the form of a nationwide lockdown was only introduced on March 25,

205

Table 1 Issues in India.

Population	1.3 billion
Literacy level	The overall literacy rate in Urban India is 79.5%
Public health expenditure	1% of GDP
Global Health Security Index rank	57 out of 195 countries in 2019
Health-care access rank	149
Health-care infrastructure adequacy rank	124
Funds allocated to the defense sector	Five times the fund allocated to health
Respiratory systems	40,000
Isolation bed	1 per 84,000 people
Doctors	1 per 11,600 patients
Hospital bed	1 per 1826 Indians

Table 2 Timeline of COVID-19 pandemic in India.

December 31, 2019	Hubei province China SARS-COVID-19
January 30	First confirmed case in India in Kerala
February 27	Final airlift from Wuhan, China (total of 759 Indians and 43 foreign nationals) and airlift from Japan (119 Indians and 5 foreign nationals)
March 6	International passenger screenings at airports
March 10 and 11	Airlift of Indians from Iran and Italy
March 12	First death secondary to COVID-19
March 13	Suspension of nonessential traveler visas
March 15	100 confirmed cases
March 22	A 1-day Janata Curfew and passenger air travel suspended till further notice
March 25	Nationwide lockdown till April 14
March 28–31	Confirmed 1 lakh cases, recovered 1 thousand cases, Cluster cases: Tablighi Jamaat
April 5	Lighted diyas
April 14	Nationwide lockdown extended till May 3
May 3	Nationwide lockdown further extended till May 31
June 1	Slow unlocking

3 months after the first COVID-19 case was reported and 2 months after the World Health Organization declared the outbreak a public health emergency of international concern. The Epidemic Disease Act[5] was implemented in entire country which allowed officials to quarantine suspected cases and close down public places. An intensive campaign was initiated, and guidelines were developed for personal hygiene, surveillance, contact tracing, quarantine, diagnosis, laboratory tests, and the management of COVID-19. All health-care facilities were asked to stop regular

outpatient and inpatient services and to continue with only emergency services. Doctors were encouraged to use telemedicine services. The Aarogya Setu app was also launched to connect essential health services with people of India to fight against COVID-19.[6] This app will inform the users of the risk, best practice, and relevant advisories pertaining to the containment of COVID-19. "Lockdown phase" was utilized by individual states to covert amenities like hotels, colleges, railway train coaches, etc. into quarantine facilities and large public places like stadiums/ trade centers were converted into isolation wards to handle an anticipated increased number of cases. Some of the states converted existing hospitals to exclusively handle COVID-19 patients. Personal protective equipment such as ventilators, face shields, and face masks production was put on priority. "Atmanirbhar program" encouraged the local experts to increase the production of necessary amenities. Time had come to prove our indigenous talent. A control room was set up at the headquarters of the General Director of Health Service to address the COVID-19 related queries. The countries of the South Asian Association for Regional Cooperation (SAARC) were invited to tackle this pandemic, and 10 million US dollars were allocated for SAARC countries.

Lockdown was extended up to May 3 and further up to May 17 and then up to May 31. Thus it was the longest lockdown (75 days) that any country has imposed in the world. Cases continue to rise even in lockdown phase, thus making us realize about community spread and the third stage of pandemic. See Fig. 1.

Definitely, lockdown has given Indians a greater chance of being alive than citizens of United Kingdom, Italy, Spain, or United States. Indian death rate in covid is 3% as compared to 5%–10% in the above-mentioned[7] countries. It gave us time for preparedness and identify the weakness and strength of this virus. The peak of pandemic in India was postponed from March–April to June, and this has enabled us to save thousands of lives.

Other measures

(1) Task force was created both at the state level and the city level. The task force updated their guidelines frequently as per recent development in treatment and local problems.

(2) Lockdown period was used to screen and identify as many cases as we can; isolate them, contact tracing, and quarantine them.

(3) Screening high-risk areas with the help of Anganwadi Sevikas or primary health workers. Without enough test kits, the 1.3-billion-person country used a gigantic surveillance network to trace and quarantine infected people.

(4) Increase the capacity of rapid testing to identify cases and isolate them. Home service of COVID-19 India's test positivity rate was 2.2% on March 22 it reached 4.7% on April 14.[8]

(5) Concentrating on production and thus increasing availability of drugs: hydroxychloroquine, tocilizumab, ivermectin, and remdesivir.

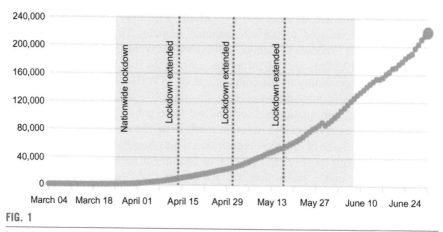

FIG. 1

Lockdown and COVID-19 active cases in India up to June 24.

Mass prophylaxis was also done for health-care workers and high-risk areas.

(6) Local classification of zone was done to segregate high-risk areas thereby preventing the spread of infection.

(7) Develop corona care facilities—COVID care center, Dedicated COVID Health Center, and Dedicated COVID Hospital.

(8) In view of increasing load of cases, home quarantine guidelines were drafted and approved by the task force.

(9) Free distribution of food grains to needy or daily wage workers. Encouraging local associations to supply food packages.

Pitfalls of our approach

This lockdown announcement was not preceded by any official planning, leading to the large-scale movement of the urban poor as they headed for their homes in rural areas. Migrants probably knew that they could be carrying the virus with them and infect their dear ones, but they desperately needed a shred of familiarity, shelter and dignity, as well as food. Some described our official strategy was an example of "too little, too late" as hidden infections were already spreading in all parts of the country, followed then by "too much, too soon" and not enough planning.

Long lockdown might be more devastating in India as it could result in economic deflection, increase hunger and poverty, and reduce public resilience to handle infection. A possibility of another peak of COVID-19 cases may occur once lockdown is lifted. A staggered unlocking of lockdown should be planned.

Future plan

Forecasting future COVID-19 pandemic is likely to take several months; social distancing and the use of masks have become important public habit. Increasing testing capacity and precautionary self-isolation of contacts is critical in reducing number of cases. Unlocking of lockdown should be done slow. Improving health-care facilities and pandemic laws to tackle future pandemic.[9] Improving telemedicine facilities, which play vital role in home quarantine facilities.[9,10] To carry fast-track research on vaccines and antibody testing for herd immunity. In any post-pandemic world, whether it is US-centric or China-centric, there is no scenario in which India, a universe in itself, and home to one-sixth of humanity, will not occupy a place. It is up to citizens: Will we emerge as part of the problem or as part of the solution? Will we emerge weaker or stronger as a nation? The pandemic has brought us to an inflection point. How we deal with it will determine our place in the future world order.

Conclusion

Pandemics have forced humans to break with the past and imagine their world anew. COVID-19 pandemic is portal, a gateway between one world and the next. We can only hope that the dark cloud of the virus sails away with the present implementation of laws and restrictions on the public. The health-care system and future proof pandemic laws ought to be given priority and must be streamlined to ensure the availability of immediate assistance even in the remotest corners of the country. Ultimately, the individual need to strive to extricate our country from this situation as advised by Krishna, "Uddharet Atmanatmanam—a person has to lift himself up; a man is his own best friend as also enemy." We as individuals should like Arjuna proclaimed "Nashto Moha—my illusion is gone." And we should stand together, do our duties, and win this "pandemic of COVID-19"

References

1. Jain VK, Iyengar K, Vaish A, Vaishy R. Differential mortality in COVID-19 patients from India and western countries. *Diabetes Metab Syndr*. 2020;14(5):1037–1041.
2. Sengupta A, Nundy S. The private health sector in India is burgeoning, but at the cost of public health care. *BMJ*. 2005;331(7526):1157–1158.
3. Government of India. *National Health Policy*; 2002. http://mohfw.nic.in/np2002.htm. Accessed 1 October 2005.
4. Reid D. India confirms its first coronavirus case. *CNBC*. 2020. Available from: https://www.cnbc.com/2020/01/30/india-confirms-first-case-of-the-coronavirus.html.
5. *Central Government Act The Epidemic Diseases Act*; 1897.
6. Singh S. Aarogya Setu is Government of India's first 'comprehensive' COVID-19 tracking app, here are all the details. *Financial Express*. 2020. April 02.

7. Chaubey G. Coronavirus (SARS-CoV-2) and mortality rate in India: the winning edge. *Front Public Health.* 2020;8:397.

8. GOVERNMENT, HEALTH, THE SCIENCES. *India's COVID-19 Testing Conundrum: Why the Govt and Critics Are Both Right*; 2020. 27 April https://science.thewire.in/health/india-covid-19-testing-contradiction-rate/.

9. Khanna RC, Cicinelli MV, Gilbert SS, Honavar SG, Murthy GSV. COVID-19 pandemic: lessons learned and future directions. *Indian J Ophthalmol.* 2020;68(5):703–710.

10. Bhaskar S, Bradley S, Chattu VK, Adisesh A, Nurtazina A. Telemedicine as the new out-patient clinic gone digital: position paper from the pandemic health system REsilience PROGRAM (REPROGRAM) international consortium (Part 2). *Front Public Health.* 2020;8:410.

Life after COVID-19: Future directions?

21

Pravin Amin

Bombay Hospital Institute of Medical Sciences, Mumbai, India

Introduction

The present-day pandemic of the severe acute respiratory syndrome coronavirus 2 (SARS-CoV-2), a novel *Betacoronavirus*, originating from Hubei Province in the People's Republic of China, has spread to 213 countries and territories around the world. This virus is a member of the Coronaviridae family, it is a highly virulent pathogenic viral infection having an incubation period between 2 and 12 days, transmitted by inhaling infected droplets or physical contact with disease-ridden droplets. On December 31, 2019, the World Health Organization (WHO) China Country Office was informed of cases of pneumonia of unknown etiology identified in Wuhan City, Hubei Province of China.[1] The virus moved from animals to humans at the Huanan Seafood Wholesale Market in Wuhan, China. The 2019 coronavirus at the whole-genome level is 96% identical to a bat coronavirus.[2] Between December 31, 2019 and January 3, 2020, a total of 44 patients with pneumonia of unknown etiology have been reported by the Chinese authorities to WHO. The Chinese isolated the virus on January 7, 2020 as a new type coronavirus, the novel SARS-CoV-2, and later shared the genetic sequence with the world so as to develop specific diagnostic kit.[3] The first fatality was noted on January 11, 2020. The Chinese New Year enhanced the spread to other provinces in China and neighboring countries like Thailand, Japan, Singapore, Vietnam, and South Korea rapidly due to movement in and out of Wuhan. WHO announced "coronavirus disease 2019 (COVID-19)" as the new name for this novel disease on February 11, 2020. During a press briefing on March 11, 2020, as the virus spread across the globe, WHO categorized COVID-19 to be a pandemic. The number of SARS-CoV-2 remaining asymptomatic has yet to be defined. Among symptomatic patients, the clinical presentation consists of fever, sore throat, anosmia, ageusia, cough, nasal congestion, fatigue, diarrhea, and features of upper respiratory tract infections.[4] In the event of serious disease, the manifestation includes severe chest discomfort with breathlessness and acute respiratory distress syndrome (ARDS). The necessity for intensive care unit admission is indicated to treat ARDS, shock, acute kidney injury, and multiple organ failure. The WHO acknowledged that in the event of mild infection, patients usually recover in about 2 weeks, with generally no complications. However, in severe or critical cases,

COVID-19 Pandemic. https://doi.org/10.1016/B978-0-323-82860-4.00001-X

patients may take 3–6 weeks to recover and may have significant morbidity and even mortality. All ages are susceptible to pick up the infection, and health-care workers (HCW) are at a higher risk. The person-to-person transmission of the COVID-19 is estimated by the reproduction number (R_0). The WHO has estimated R_0 to be between 1.4 and 2.5,[5] whereas others have estimated R_0 to be between 2.0 and 3.3.[6] The basic case reproduction rate is probably between 2 and 6.47.[5] The treatment is largely symptomatic and supportive; when patients get hypoxic, oxygen is provided with either nasal prongs, face or venturi mask, or non-rebreathing masks. In patients who are more hypoxic, the high-flow nasal cannula or noninvasive ventilation may be used, and in the critical patients, elective invasive ventilation is indicated. Drugs with antiviral properties such as ribavirin, lopinavir-ritonavir, favipiravir, ivermectin, nitazoxanide combination of azithromycin, and hydroxychloroquine have not yielded very satisfactory results. Remdesivir a broad-spectrum antiviral agent used against Ebola has shown benefits in the treatment of COVID-19.[7] Various immunomodulators such as IL-6 inhibitor (e.g., tocilizumab, sarilumab) have been used when inflammatory markers (e.g., D-dimer, ferritin) and pro-inflammatory cytokines such as interleukin IL-6 are elevated in severe COVID-19.[8] The belief is that by using these immunomodulators, disease progression may be prevented. The use of low-dose dexamethasone in a large trial in the United Kingdom reduced deaths by 35% in ventilated patients.[9] Convalescent plasma may be of benefit if given in the early phase of the mild-to-moderate form of the disease, but this form of therapy currently remains unclear.[10]

Earlier pandemics

Three of the deadliest pandemics as recorded in history were caused by a bacterium, *Yersinia pestis*, leading to a fatal infection otherwise known as the plague. The Plague of Justinian arrived in Constantinople, the capital of the Byzantine Empire (541–549 CE). It was carried over by ships across the Mediterranean Sea from Egypt by grain and plague-ridden fleas on black rats. The plague annihilated Constantinople and spread all across Europe, Asia, North Africa, and the Arab killing approximately 30–50 million people, nearly half of the world's population. The plague really never left, and when it came back about 800 years later, it caused devastation. When Europe was hit in 1347 by the Black Death, more than 200 million lives were claimed in just 4 years. The etiology was later discovered by Alexandre Yersin from the Institut Pasteur, while investigating the plague epidemic in the year 1894 in Hong Kong.[11] The cholera pandemics occurred all through the 19th century, a minimum of six widespread outbreaks of cholera was documented but may have been much more. It started in India in the Bay of Bengal region and was responsible for tens of thousands of deaths. The Influenza virus was also responsible for large fatalities in various pandemics. The first significant flu pandemic the Russian Flu of 1889 started in Siberia spread to Moscow, from there it spread to the rest of Europe. In the subsequent year, it moved to North America and Africa, over 360,000 died. The Spanish flu of 1918 is likely the worst pandemic of the 20th century, the

1918 flu infected up to one-third of the global population and killed up to 50 million people. At that time, the causative agent was unknown, but the cause was later detected in 1930. Reviewing historical publications indicated the presence of bacterial coinfections which perhaps contributed to the high mortality during that era. On February 1957, a new avian influenza A (H2N2) virus emerged in East Asia, sparking a pandemic the so-called "Asian Flu." A second wave followed in early 1958, causing an approximate 1.1 million deaths globally. The smallpox caused devastation in the 20th century leading to between 300 million and 500 million deaths. The WHO reported till as recent as 1967 that about 15 million people become infected with the disease and that nearly 2 million died that year. The Plague of Athens that occurred in 430 BCE, and the Antonine Plague, which spread to the Roman Empire in 165–180 CE, may have been caused by smallpox. Human immunodeficiency virus (HIV) pandemic was identified in 1981,[12] acquired immunodeficiency syndrome (AIDS) was first observed in American gay communities but is believed to have developed from a chimpanzee virus from West Africa. This disease which spreads through body fluids has affected over 38 million cases of HIV worldwide. Of this, 24 million people are undergoing antiretroviral therapy. About 32 million people have died due to AIDS since the onset of the disease. The first influenza pandemic of the 21st century occurred in 2009–2010 and was caused by an influenza A (H1N1) virus. It was likely that 1,51,700–5,75,400 cardiovascular and respiratory deaths was connected with 2009 influenza A H1N1 pandemic in the first year of the illness in every country in the world. The 21st century saw four epidemics of concern: SARS-CoV, Ebola, Middle East respiratory syndrome (MERS), and Zika. Of these, two SARS and MERS are related to the current pandemic as both these diseases are caused due to coronaviruses. SARS-CoV or SARS-CoV-1 was first identified in 2003, SARS-CoV-1 is believed to have possibly started from bats, spread to cats, and then to humans in China, followed by spreading to 26 other countries, infecting 8096 people, with 774 deaths.[13] MERS or camel flu can be a fatal respiratory illness caused by a betacoronavirus (MERS-CoV). Most cases of MERS have occurred in Saudi Arabia and the United Arab Emirates but has spread to Asia, Europe, and America. Both these diseases have clinical presentations similar to COVID-19. SARS-CoV-2 like SARS-CoV-1 acts on the same human cell receptor, the angiotensin-converting enzyme 2 (ACE-2), while MERS-CoV uses dipeptidyl peptidase-4 to enter into the host cells. The R_0 of COVID-19 is estimated by WHO to range between 2 and 2.5, which is higher than that for SARS-CoV-1 (1.7–1.9) and MERS (<1), clearly indicating that SARS-CoV-2 has a higher potential of pandemic as opposed to SARS-CoV-1 and MERS. The fatality rate of COVID-19 infection is projected to be 2.3%, which is lower than SARS-CoV-1 (9.5%) and clearly much lower than MERS (34.4%).[14] An important experience learnt from the coronaviruses is the high frequency of HCW being affected by infected patients more so during aerosol-generating procedures (AGP), such as sneezing, coughing, cardiopulmonary resuscitation, intubation, and tracheostomy. In Toronto, 13% of HCW involved in intubations acquired SARS during SARS-CoV-1.[15] In the same pandemic in Singapore, 40% of HCW developed nosocomial SARS-CoV-1 and 6% of HCW's died.[16]

Lessons learnt from previous pandemics

In the 1850s, the cities like London, New York, and Paris rebuilt their sewage systems following a century-long global cholera pandemic that killed over 1.5 million people which piloted in a modern urban public health that spread across the world. In 1900 following a typhoid epidemic in the city of Chicago, the city engineers reversed the flow of the river in Chicago, as a result terminating the adulteration of Lake Michigan, which was the principal source of drinking water for the city.

Nonpharmaceutical interventions

During the Spanish Flu, numerous nonpharmaceutical approaches were commissioned to limit the spread of virus and to treat patients. Some of these measures are important and applicable in current and future outbreaks, epidemics, and even pandemics.

Quarantine

The exercise of implementing quarantine, began in the 14th century to safeguard coastal towns from plague epidemics. The dockyards in Venice required ships to set anchor for 40 days before being allowed to dock. This was termed quarantine and was derived from two Italian words *"quaranta giorni"* which stands for 40 days. The concept of quarantine may have preceded the Black Death, as the practice of isolating the sick, dates back to earlier times, and is referred to in the Bible with respect to segregating people with leprosy. Australia enacted maritime quarantine both in the first and initial part of second wave. This initial quarantine safeguarded Australia from the second wave of the pandemic till December 1918, this was when quarantine was infringed.[17] Air travel has revolutionized global travel as opposed to earlier maritime transport in the last century. This is in fact why there is rapid spread across international borders in the influenza pandemics in 1957, 1968, and 2009.[18] However, in 2009, airport authorities used modern techniques to screen passengers arriving from potential areas of the outbreak. This method of screening on arrival of international passengers is not likely to prevent the spread of airborne or droplet infections.

Large gatherings

In most cities during the 1918 pandemic, simple nonpharmaceutical methods were implemented to prevent person-to-person spread of the flu. This would involve closing down auditoriums, places of worship, schools, funerals, processions, weddings, and large gatherings so as to prevent crowds and build the concept of social distancing.[19] In Hong Kong during the 2009 influenza pandemic, a 25% reduction transmission of the flu was noted after schools were closed for a month.[20]

Lockdown

The efficacy of a lockdown to counter the pandemic of COVID-19 has mixed views, the political argument seems to have negative impact by tanking the national economy. The skeptics would question a compromise between protecting a society's health or damage the economy. Countries like Taiwan controlled the outbreak without imposing a lockdown, whereas China implemented a strict lockdown and was able to contain the spread of the virus. Sweden on the other hand did not implement a lockdown but put into action a reverse quarantine by protecting the elderly and highly susceptible individuals with comorbidities, The United States of America implemented a lockdown in areas with high contagion but lifted it very early. The United Kingdom like Sweden opted for the concept of herd immunity but quickly implemented lockdown as numbers started to soar. India like many other Asian countries implemented a preemptive lockdown when the numbers of COVID-19 was low; however, after nearly 40 days of lockdown under severe economic crisis, the government reluctantly lifted the lockdown prematurely and continued regional lockdown based on district-wise resurgence of the contagion. In a cross-country analysis, of lockdown measures more so with the European model, its effectiveness begins in about 3 weeks after implementing the lockdown and number of COVID-19 infections keeps on reducing for as much as 20 days.

Hygiene

Handwashing with soap and water has been advocated from time immemorial and has been documented in studies by Ignaz Semmelweis in Vienna in the mid-1800s to reduce infections. Frequent handwashing has been known to limit the spread of the influenza virus during the 1918 pandemic, this was primarily due to influenza viruses being transmitted because of hand-to-face contact. In influenza pandemics, comparing the frequency of handwashing with laboratory-confirmed influenza found a significant protective effect while analyzing the available data.[21] Handwashing with antibacterial solutions did not extend any benefit over soap and water. In Hong Kong during the SARS-CoV-1 outbreak in a case–control study, handwashing over ten times in a day and disinfecting fomites in a multivariate analysis was shown to be protective.[22] The concepts of respiratory hygiene and cough etiquette involve using source control measures to prevent patients with respiratory infections from transmitting their infections to others. Persons with respiratory symptoms should cover nose and mouth with a disposable tissue while coughing or sneezing followed by hand hygiene. Alternatively, cover the nose and mouth with one's elbow during the process of sneezing and coughing. People with respiratory symptoms should maintain a distance of over 3 ft from other people and should be encouraged to wear a mask.

Face masks

Before the year 1910, the usage of face protection was infrequent during any surgical procedure in hospitals. The use of surgical mask in operating rooms in the United States and Germany started around the 1920s. In the year 1940s, both washable and sterilizable masks came into vogue. In the mid-1960s, disposable masks were introduced across the globe. A surgical mask also known as a medical mask, it is essentially a loosely fitting disposable mask that protects the individual's mouth and nose from splashes, sprays, and droplets that may include microorganisms. A surgical mask may protect others in the vicinity by diminishing the spread of respiratory secretions of the person wearing the mask. A N95 mask offers more protection than a surgical mask does as it can filter out both large and small particles. The N95 mask must meet standards set by National Institute for Occupational Safety and Health, implying it needs to filter at least 95% of the particles. Some of the N95 masks have valves, this makes breathing easier. All healthcare workers (HCW) should be trained to conduct a fit test so as to ascertain a proper seal before using an N95 respirator in an infected zone. All surgical masks and N95 masks are proposed to be disposable. However, as there may be a short supply during a pandemic, some of these masks may be reused after subjecting them to sterilization. The free flight phase 2 respirators of the European Union and KN95 respirators of China are considered equivalent to N95 respirators. The evidence if N95 respirators are more effective than medical masks in preventing viral respiratory infection in HCW, is uncertain but has been shown to be protective under laboratory conditions. Some studies and systemic reviews have asserted its efficacy, while some have not.[23–25] The P100 mask protects people from particles 0.3 μm or larger and filters out all odors, making it undetectable to the human nose. A N95 mask keeps out at least 95% of particles but isn't oil resistant, and a P100 mask is oil proof while protecting the wearer from at least 99.8% of particles. P100 or high-efficiency particulate air (HEPA) filters are considered much safer than the N95 masks. While surgical and N95 masks may be in short supply and should be set aside for HCW's, cloth masks are easier to get, can be washed, and reused. This may be used by citizens in countries where wearing masks is mandatory.

Powered air purifying respirators

The powered air purifying respirators (PAPRs) have a battery that uses a blower to drive air through filter cartridges or canisters under pressure to a hood or face piece or a helmet, providing a higher assigned protection factor. The high positive pressure inside the facepiece reduces leakage in, from the external contaminated air. PAPRs have a higher protection more so during intubation and tracheostomy. They filter 99.97% of 0.3 μm sized particle and is oil proof.[26]

Personal protective equipment

The recommended personal protective equipment (PPE) for HCW caring for critically ill COVID-19 patients includes fluid-resistant gown or a hazmat suit, two pairs of long gloves, eye protection goggles, which should include side shields. Face shields can offer both eye protection and will prevent infectivity of both face and mask. Disposable shoe covers may be needed before putting on the leggings of

PPE or even the hazmat suit. Shoes should be waterproof and be capable of being disinfected. All HCW should wear scrub suits under the PPE. The PPE should be so designed for easy removal so as to avoid any blemish during removal. Hand hygiene should be carried out both during and after removing the PPE. The process of donning and doffing of PPE should be done in a stepwise fashion and ideally under the supervision of a colleague to avoid errors.

Air handling units with negative pressure

An isolation facility aims to control the airflow in the room so that the number of airborne infectious particles is reduced to a level that there is no cross infection to other people within a health-care facility. Heating, ventilation, and air-conditioning system maintain good air quality within the intensive care unit. This is an important nonpharmacological strategy to prevent nosocomial infections. WHO suggests in COVID-19 patients to be isolated in an adequately ventilated negative pressure rooms with a minimum of 12 air changes per hour, specially if AGP is intended.[27] If the air is recirculated, then the incoming air should be filtered. High-efficiency filters like HEPA filters improve the efficiency but are very expensive to maintain. HEPA filters are 99.97% efficient for removing particles with a size of $\geq 0.3\,\mu$m in diameter.

Most of these nonpharmaceutical interventions are lessons learnt from previous outbreaks and are pearls of wisdom acquired across generations. The more recent interventions improvised during recent pandemics help in limiting and suppressing an ongoing contagion.

Sequela from COVID-19

Survivors from the current pandemic may have specific organ dysfunction following infection, leading to long-term morbidity and mortality. During the SARS-CoV-1 epidemic, observational studies demonstrated that some survivors developed pulmonary fibrosis, restrictive lung anomalies, associated with impaired effort tolerance, and poor quality of life. The computed tomography scan images showed pulmonary fibrosis with air trapping and the evidence of bronchiectasis.[28] Since there are several parallels linking SARS-CoV-2 and SARS-CoV-1 infections, it is possible that lung fibrosis may be seen as long-term outcome in COVID-19 pneumonia. Pulmonary fibrotic disease has been observed in COVID-19, following pneumonia and severe ARDS. On autopsy of fatal cases, COVID-19 have demonstrated pulmonary fibrosis with evidence of severe fibrotic organizing pneumonia.[29] There is thus justification for using antifibrotic therapy and is being currently investigated.[29] During the SARS-CoV-1 epidemic, cardiac manifestations were hypotension, arrhythmias, myocarditis, and sudden cardiac arrests. MERS too was coupled with heart failure and myocarditis. COVID-19 infection may have similar cardiac signs may also be due to a direct cardiac infection by SARS-CoV-2. ACE-2 is bound to the membrane of the cell in the lungs, immune, and cardiovascular systems. ACE-2 has been identified as a functional receptor for coronaviruses. The SARS-CoV-2 infection is initiated by the spike protein of the virus attaching to ACE2, which then more so in the heart and lungs manifest its clinical presentation.[30] During the SARS-CoV-1 epidemic often ended up having hyperlipidemia, cardiovascular disease or diabetes mellitus on long-term follow-up.[31] As the coronaviruses are similar, patients recovering from COVID-19 too need to be followed up for these conditions. In COVID-19, liver injury may be due to the direct invasion of the virus into the liver cells or due to drug-induced liver injury and or from the cytokine storm or even due to severe hypoxic injury.[32] However, long-term manifestations will need to be monitored. In the central nervous system, altered mental status due to encephalopathy or encephalitis and primary psychiatric presentation is usually seen in younger patients.[33] Clinical presentations vary from headache, seizure, encephalitis, strokes with vascular events, and even Guillain-Barré syndrome.[34] Long-term manifestations are yet to be reported.

Economic impact

The COVID-19 pandemic is bringing huge economic, social, and health-care challenges. As per the international monetary fund (IMF), the global economy is projected to decline by over 4.9% at the end of 2020. There will be a precipitous slowdown ever since the Great Depression in the 1930s. The COVID-19 pandemic has thrust the economy around the globe into a tail spin, leading to the financial system shrinking with cessation of growth. In the United States, ever since COVID-19 pandemic surfaced in the month of April, over 20.5 million have lost their jobs. The IMF has said the global economy will take a $12 trillion hit from the COVID-19 pandemic, it would take 2 years for world output to return to levels at the end of 2019. The COVID-19 pandemic thrusted economies into a great lockdown, which hindered the spread of the virus and saved lives but additionally sparked the worst recession since the Great Depression. The manufacturing productivity has dipped considerably in many countries, essentially due to a decrease in demand. China's gross domestic product (GDP) plummeted by 36.6% in the first quarter of 2020, but South Korea, which did not impose a lockdown but followed a strategy of aggressive testing, contact tracing, and quarantining, had a drop in output of 5.5%. World's topmost economies such as the USA, China, UK, Germany, France, Italy, Japan, and many others are at the verge of collapse. The travel, tourism, hospitality, and industry has been decimated by the pandemic. Oil prices have fallen to an all-time low, and the transport sector, which consumes 60% of the oil utilization, has been affected as numerous countries imposed lockdowns. During the lockdown, prices of foodstuff and grocery had increased affecting common people. Extending lockdowns has huge economic impacts on people in the low-income and at-risk categories. High income countries have rolled out finance packages. While India's economic stimulus package was 10% of its GDP, Japan's economic package was 21.1%, the USA 13%, Sweden 12%, Germany 10.7%, France 9.3%, Spain 7.3%, and Italy 5.7%. South Korea and Taiwan economies were hardly affected as they did not stop their businesses during the outbreak in their countries. China, which lifted its lockdown after controlling the contagion, has been gradually reopening its economy without encountering a second wave of infection. Lockdowns have led to cleaner cities and a reduction in greenhouse gas emissions.[35]

Climate change and pandemics

There are clear connections between COVID-19 and the climate crisis. Though the virus is believed to have originated with the horseshoe bat, they have been living in the forests of the globe for 40 million years and flourishes in the remote jungles of south China. Researcher have shown that pollution worsens the outcome of COVID-19 patients as seen in New York and Milan, two very densely populated cities. COVID-19 could well be nature's warning against climate change as 2019 observed shocking heat waves in Europe, record wildfires in Australia, large number of deaths due to cyclones, and a large number of severe weather conditions. The last 5 years were the warmest on record, and the frequency and intensity of natural disasters are on the rise. The question is, Did these climate changes trigger the pandemic? Though this may not be proven to be so, but history indicates that certain outbreaks are directly or indirectly linked to climate change. It is noteworthy that over the last 15 years, climate change has increased the outbreaks of malaria, dengue, Zika, West Nile virus, Nipah valley virus, and Ebola. Deforestation is linked to 31% of disease outbreaks such as the Ebola, Zika, and Nipah viruses. Roughly 70% of new pathogens come from animals and about 30% of these is ascribed to deforestation, establishing farming near these forests, utilization of natural resource. One study estimates that more than 3200 strains of coronaviruses already exist among bats, awaiting an opportunity to jump to people.[36] Researchers at the Tibetan Plateau in China demonstrated that since thousands of years, they have demonstrated in the glacier viruses, most of these are unknown in the virology dataset. The researchers showed 33 groups of these virus species in the ice glaciers, of these some are potentially pathogenic.

Medications in a pandemic

In general, most cases of COVID-19, there is clearly no need for antiviral therapy and most patients can be managed by supportive care. The SARS-CoV-1 pandemic which appeared unexpectedly in 2003 quickly spread to other countries leaving the medical world in significant distress. Potential therapies were explored based on in vitro studies, without adequate randomized trials, these drugs were fast-tracked into therapy for these sick patients. Some sense was found later from observational cohort studies and case reports. Yet, this data was beneficial in offering clinical guidelines and giving future direction to research in case similar outbreaks reappears. Early in the SARS-CoV-1 pandemic, a combination of ribavirin and corticosteroids were used, so lopinavir/ritonavir too was used. Interferon-alpha, an antiviral used to treat a broad spectrum of viruses, seemed to work against SARS in cell culture tests and was tried in some patients. Like seasonal flu, most people recovered from the H1N1 2009 pandemic usually within a week, without any antiviral medications. Antiviral agents prevent, shorten, and reduce the severity of flu. Antiviral agents used for the treatment and prevention of H1N1 are oseltamivir and zanamivir, but amantadine and rimantadine were ineffective, in severe cases steroids were used. In the Ebola epidemic in 2014, a large number of people developed Ebola viral infection in western Africa; several therapies were administered against the virus, this included chloroquine and its derivative hydroxychloroquine, favipiravir, monoclonal antibodies, and convalescent plasma. In general, most cases of COVID-19, there is clearly no need for antiviral therapy, and most patients can be managed by supportive care. Frequently used antiviral drugs against the current virus in this pandemic are listed in Table 1. Other agents like immunomodulating agents that prevent hyperinflammation due to cytokine storm has been used. Interleukin inhibitors like tocilizumab may prevent severe damage to lung parenchyma due to the cytokine release in cases of severe COVID-19 infections.[8] The use of 10 days of dexamethasone in COVID-19 patients had an excellent outcome both in survival and limiting duration on ventilators.[9] Currently, there are no highly effective broad-spectrum antiviral

Table 1 Drugs with potential antiviral properties tried in cases of Covid-19.

Drug groups	Drugs	Dose
Viral entry inhibitors	Hydroxychloroquine Chloroquine	Days 1–5: 2 × 200 mg/day, orally
Inhibitors of viral protein synthesis	Lopinavir/ritonavir	Days 1–10 (or 14): 400 mg/ 100 mg × 2/day, orally
Inhibitors of viral RNA polymerase/RNA synthesis	Remdesivir	Day 1: 200 mg, IV Days 2–5 (or 10): 100 mg/day, IV
	Favipiravir	Day 1: 2 × 1600 mg Days 2–7 (or 10): 2 × 600 mg/day
Immunomodulators	Nitazoxanide	Nitazoxanide 500 mg twice daily orally with meal for 6 days
	Ivermectin	Ivermectin 200 µg/kg once orally on an empty stomach
Immune Interferon	IFN-α	IFN-α is vapor inhalation at a dose of 5 million U for adults, 2 times/day
Guanosine analogue inhibits synthesis of viral mRNA	Ribavirin	IV infusion at a dose of 500 mg for adults, 2–3 times/day
Dual-acting direct antiviral/host-targeting agent	Arbidol	200 mg, 3 times/day
Antirhinoviral macrolides of antiviral gene mRNA and protein	Azithromycin	500 mg OD × 5 days

agents, or specific agents capable of interrupting viral life cycle, or destroying receptor proteins on the virus. Theoretically, monoclonal antibodies generally bind to specific proteins. These antibodies provide passive immunization against specific portion of the virus so as to reduce the multiplication of the virus and limit the severity of the illness. In the ideal world, neutralize the virus with the monoclonal antibody till an appropriate vaccine is generated against the contagion.[37]

Vaccines

Edward Jenner invented a method to protect against smallpox in the 18th century. After observing that cowpox infection seemed to protect humans against smallpox, he observed that milkmaids who previously had caught cowpox did not catch smallpox. At the end of late 1940s, large-scale vaccine production was conceived, and disease control was set in motion. The next array of vaccines was discovered and produced in the early part of the 20th century. These were vaccines against pertussis in 1914, diphtheria in 1926, and tetanus in 1938. These set of vaccines were then merged together in 1948 and became the DTP vaccine. Jonas Salk invented the polio vaccine which was then licensed in 1955. In 1963, the measles vaccine was developed, and at the late 1960s, vaccines were also available to protect against mumps in 1967 and rubella in 1969. These three vaccines were then combined into the MMR vaccine in 1971. Vaccine that was developed in the 1980s included hepatitis B and *Haemophilus influenzae* type b. New vaccines developed later include varicella (1996), hepatitis A (2000), pneumococcal vaccine (2001), rotavirus (2008), hepatitis A (2006), human papillomavirus (2011), and meningococcal serogroup B vaccine (2014).

The influenza virus was detected in 1933 leading rapidly to the development of the first-generation live-attenuated vaccines. The first ever monovalent inactivated flu vaccine was of influenza A. After finding the influenza B virus, the bivalent vaccine was available on 1942. The first trivalent vaccine consisted of two types of influenza A strains, and one strain of influenza B was available for administration on 1978. Since 1940, researchers have demonstrated that there has been a successive drift in the strains altering the antigenicity in the virus and hence the vaccine has often been altered to mirror these changes. Future vaccines will need to be modified to adapt to changes in strains. During this illness, there is a rapid research in developing a vaccine for COVID-19, but it may already be too late to impact the outcome of the first wave in this pandemic. There are numerous potential vaccines currently undergoing clinical trials yet to provide many meaningful results. This fight against coronaviruses (SARS-CoV-1 and MERS-CoV) may not be simple as the previous two coronaviruses did not yield favorable results. In 2003–2004, numerous SARS-CoV-1 vaccines made it to phase I clinical trials and did not move up into further phases as eradication of the virus by nonpharmaceutical methods materialized. Inactivated virus vaccine and a spike-based DNA vaccine had proved to be safe and possibly generated neutralizing antibodies.

For Covid-19 currently there are seven distinctive vaccines across three platforms that have been developed and are in use across different countries. The most vulnerable populations in large number of countries have been vaccinated in the early part of 2021. Two messenger RNA (mRNA) vaccines are currently available one developed by Pfizer (BNT162b2) and the other one being by Moderna (mRNA-1273). Once injected, the mRNA is seized by macrophages which then produce spike protein. The spike protein is then presented on the surface of these macrophages, leading to formation of antibodies against the spike proteins and renders protection against the SARS-CoV-2 infection. The enzymes within the body then destroy and dispose of the mRNA. In this vaccine, no live virus is included. There are four nonreplicating vector vaccines. (1) ChAdOx1-S recombinant vaccine is a chimpanzee-derived adenovirus vaccine developed by University of Oxford and AstraZeneca. This "vector" virus is the virus that causes common cold and not COVID-19. This vector virus which is present within the vaccine produces the SARS-CoV-2 spike protein. (2) Ad26.COV2.S, is an Ad26-vector, is a nonreplicating adenoviral vector vaccine against coronavirus disease, the vaccine conceived by Janssen and known as Johnson & Johnson single dose vaccine. (3) Sputnik V developed by Gamaleya, designed from two different adenoviral vectors Ad26 and Ad5 producing antibodies to spike protein. (4) Ad5-nCoV created by CanSino Biologics in China, where an Ad5 vector is used to express the spike protein antibody. There are other inactivated vaccines and nasal vaccines in phase 3 trials currently underway in India and China. More than 60 vaccines are in clinical development, but challenges faced by governments is to build up manufacturing capabilities to fulfil the needs of general population. Vaccines are a critical new tool in the battle against COVID-19 and it is immensely reassuring to see so many vaccines proving to be successful and getting developed.[38]

Planning for future pandemics

In the two decades of the 21st century, mankind has faced a number of pandemics (SARS-CoV-1, 2009 H1N1 influenza, 2013 chikungunya, SARS-CoV-2) and epidemics (2006 chikungunya, meningitis, cholera, measles, yellow fever, Zika, and MERS). In every outbreak, the nature of pathogen poses challenges to public health system more so in low- and middle-income countries. Health for all is the basic and fundamental right for all human beings. At times of outbreaks, epidemics, and pandemics, the world looks forward to the WHO to take a leadership role and provides solutions to the ongoing outbreak. Since the WHO was founded back in 1948, it has taken leadership roles in major medical emergencies across the globe. It has done a stellar job over the years but has been found wanting in some situations, more so during the Ebola outbreak.[39] Over the years, there are concerns regarding funding for the WHO, which does come to the fore during budget spending for perceived outbreaks and threats. In major crisis, WHO needs to interact and share strategies with other similar organizations like Centers for Disease Control and Prevention (CDC), Collation for Epidemic Preparedness Innovations, and the Global Research Collaboration for Infectious Disease Preparedness. This coordination between organizations will help in preventing duplication and cutting costs. Most outbreaks and acute public health risks are generally unpredictable and need well-directed strategies. In 2005, the International Health Regulations (IHR) provided a central legal charter that defined countries rights and commitments in dealing with public health incidents and emergencies that can potentially cross international borders. The IHR is legally binding on 196 countries, this includes the 194 WHO Member States. The Joint External Evaluation Tool of the IHR is able to assess a country's capacity to prevent, detect, and rapidly respond to public health threats independently.[40] The greatest tests to achieve control during an outbreak is arranging a trained personnel with the required skill in clinical management, public health, epidemiology, and numerous specialities in the field of medicine. Civic bodies while planning for large epidemics and pandemics delegate teams to meet the mandatory surge capacity encountered following the contagion. This involves trained human HCW's, physical structures able to accommodate hospital beds, and appropriate medical gear and equipment. In the current pandemic, cities across India were able to convert auditoriums, stadiums wedding halls into large medical facilities, but these centres were run with skeletal staff making the logistics truly very trying but did take a load of some of the active medical facilities. In hospitals, elective surgeries were canceled making way for more hospital beds to address the contagion. The financial implications of limiting elective work may have deleterious effects on the financial model of these institutes. Countries which generally do well during outbreaks are those nations which have both robust preventive public health systems and excellent curative health services. During an outbreak, the absolute numbers open doors for potential research and are capable of generating the numbers to get meaningful outcomes in diagnostics and therapeutics. Large information too can be collected prospectively in observational studies to elicit consequential data. Finally, vigorous infection control measures have to be spread to HCW and community too; as in this pandemic, the most susceptible individuals are colleagues at work and immediate family members. In recent times, there has been a surge in global terrorism, the possibility of a contagion being used as a bioterrorism apparatus is a distinct possibility the nations must remain vigilant against this lurking threat. In 1975, a Biological Weapons Convention ensured an embargo on the production and utilization of biological weapons. Over 180 countries participated in the convention and endorsed the proceedings. Terrorist organizations and nation that support them do not follow the established rules and are potentially a huge threat if biological weapons are used against susceptible nations.[41]

Conclusion

This century has already seen numerous outbreaks, epidemics, and pandemic, having a major impact on health care, huge economic impacts affecting the livelihoods of ordinary people increasing mortality in highly susceptible individuals. Organizations like the WHO and CDC have laid down protocols and guidelines to be implemented during outbreaks, these etiquettes need to be implemented in its full propriety to avert and minimize risk to human beings. Across affected countries, the biggest impact has been on large crowded cities leading to lockdowns. Lockdowns lead to prolonged cutbacks in commercial activity from, lockdowns will hit low-income and susceptible factions the hardest. World leaders more so from the developed nations need to address the clear and present danger a pandemic that exposes the free world. These nation-states need to plan for future contagion and the possible impacts it can have on health and the economies of the world. In the current COVID-19 pandemic, Bill Gates quoted "In any crisis leaders have two equally important responsibilities: solve the immediate problem and keep it from happening again." However, well we prepare, some storms will have a significant toll. The final answer in the event of an outbreak happens is to ensure a rapid development of vaccines.

References

1. WHO. *Pneumonia of Unknown Cause – China*. World Heal Organization; 2020. https://www.who.int/csr/don/05-january-2020-pneumonia-of-unkown-cause-china/en/.
2. Zhou P, Yang XL, Wang XG, et al. A pneumonia outbreak associated with a new coronavirus of probable bat origin. *Nature*. 2020;579(7798):270–273.
3. Wang C, Horby PW, Hayden FG, Gao GF. A novel coronavirus outbreak of global health concern. *Lancet*. 2020;395(10223):470–473.
4. Guan WJ, Ni ZY, Hu Y, et al. Clinical characteristics of coronavirus disease 2019 in China. *N Engl J Med*. 2020;382(18):1708–1720.
5. Cheng ZJ, Shan J. 2019 novel coronavirus: where we are and what we know. *Infection*. 2020;48(2):155–163.
6. Majumder MS, Mandl KD. Early in the epidemic: impact of preprints on global discourse about COVID-19 transmissibility. *Lancet Glob Health*. 2020;8(5):e627–e630.
7. Beigel JH, Tomashek KM, Dodd LE, et al. Remdesivir for the treatment of covid-19 preliminary report. *N Engl J Med*. 2020.
8. Jordan SC, Zakowski P, Tran HP, et al. Compassionate use of tocilizumab for treatment of SARS-CoV-2 pneumonia. *Clin Infect Dis*. 2020.
9. Horby PLW, Emberson J, RECOVERY Collaborative Group. Effect of dexamethasone in hospitalized patients with COVID-19: preliminary report. *medRxiv*. 2020. https://doi.org/10.1101/2020.06.22.20137273.
10. Joyner MJ, Wright RS, Fairweather D, et al. Early safety indicators of COVID-19 convalescent plasma in 5,000 patients. *J Clin Invest*. 2020;130(9):4791–4797.
11. Drancourt M, Raoult D. Molecular history of plague. *Clin Microbiol Infect*. 2016;22(11):911–915.
12. Cohen MS, Hellmann N, Levy JA, DeCock K, Lange J. The spread, treatment, and prevention of HIV-1: evolution of a global pandemic. *J Clin Invest*. 2008;118(4):1244–1254.
13. WHO. *Summary of Probable SARS Cases with Onset of Illness from 1 November 2002 to 31 July 2003*; 2004. http://www.who.int/csr/sars/country/table2004_04_21/en/index.html.
14. Petrosillo N, Viceconte G, Ergonul O, Ippolito G, Petersen E. COVID-19, SARS and MERS: are they closely related? *Clin Microbiol Infect*. 2020;26(6):729–734.
15. Caputo KM, Byrick R, Chapman MG, Orser BJ, Orser BA. Intubation of SARS patients: infection and perspectives of healthcare workers. *Can J Anaesth*. 2006;53(2):122–129.

16. Oh VM, Lim TK. Singapore's experience of SARS. *Clin Med (Lond)*. 2003;3(5):448–451.
17. Shanks GD, Wilson N, Kippen R, Brundage JF. The unusually diverse mortality patterns in the Pacific region during the 1918-21 influenza pandemic: reflections at the pandemic's centenary. *Lancet Infect Dis*. 2018;18(10):e323–e332.
18. Khan K, Arino J, Hu W, et al. Spread of a novel influenza A (H1N1) virus via global airline transportation. *N Engl J Med*. 2009;361(2):212–214.
19. Bootsma MC, Ferguson NM. The effect of public health measures on the 1918 influenza pandemic in U.S. cities. *Proc Natl Acad Sci U S A*. 2007;104(18):7588–7593.
20. Wu JT, Cowling BJ, Lau EH, et al. School closure and mitigation of pandemic (H1N1) 2009. *Hong Kong Emerg Infect Dis*. 2010;16(3):538–541.
21. Cheng VC, Tai JW, Wong LM, et al. Prevention of nosocomial transmission of swine-origin pandemic influenza virus A/H1N1 by infection control bundle. *J Hosp Infect*. 2010;74(3):271–277.
22. World Health Organization Writing G, Bell D, Nicoll A, et al. Non-pharmaceutical interventions for pandemic influenza, national and community measures. *Emerg Infect Dis*. 2006;12(1):88–94.
23. Smith JD, MacDougall CC, Johnstone J, Copes RA, Schwartz B, Garber GE. Effectiveness of N95 respirators versus surgical masks in protecting health care workers from acute respiratory infection: a systematic review and meta-analysis. *CMAJ*. 2016;188(8):567–574.
24. Offeddu V, Yung CF, Low MSF, Tam CC. Effectiveness of masks and respirators against respiratory infections in healthcare workers: a systematic review and meta-analysis. *Clin Infect Dis*. 2017;65(11):1934–1942.
25. Radonovich Jr LJ, Simberkoff MS, Bessesen MT, et al. N95 respirators vs medical masks for preventing influenza among health care personnel: a randomized clinical trial. *JAMA*. 2019;322(9):824–833.
26. Ha JF. The COVID-19 pandemic, personal protective equipment and respirator: a narrative review. *Int J Clin Pract*. 2020;74:e13578.
27. WHO. *Infection Prevention and Control During Health Care When COVID-19 Is Suspected: Interim Guidance, 19 March 2020*; 2020. https://apps.who.int/iris/handle/10665/331495.
28. Hui DS, Wong KT, Ko FW, et al. The 1-year impact of severe acute respiratory syndrome on pulmonary function, exercise capacity, and quality of life in a cohort of survivors. *Chest*. 2005;128(4):2247–2261.
29. George PM, Wells AU, Jenkins RG. Pulmonary fibrosis and COVID-19: the potential role for antifibrotic therapy. *Lancet Respir Med*. 2020.
30. Zheng YY, Ma YT, Zhang JY, Xie X. COVID-19 and the cardiovascular system. *Nat Rev Cardiol*. 2020;17(5):259–260.
31. Wu Q, Zhou L, Sun X, et al. Altered lipid metabolism in recovered SARS patients twelve years after infection. *Sci Rep*. 2017;7(1):9110.
32. Zhang C, Shi L, Wang FS. Liver injury in COVID-19: management and challenges. *Lancet Gastroenterol Hepatol*. 2020;5(5):428–430.
33. Varatharaj A, Thomas N, Ellul MA, et al. Neurological and neuropsychiatric complications of COVID-19 in 153 patients: a UK-wide surveillance study. *Lancet Psychiatry*. 2020;7(10):875–882.
34. Zubair AS, McAlpine LS, Gardin T, Farhadian S, Kuruvilla DE, Spudich S. Neuropathogenesis and neurologic manifestations of the coronaviruses in the age of coronavirus disease 2019: a review. *JAMA Neurol*. 2020;77(8):1018–1027.

35. The Lancet Planetary Health. Post-COVID-19 spending. *Lancet Planet Health*. 2020;4 (5):e168.

36. Tang XC, Zhang JX, Zhang SY, et al. Prevalence and genetic diversity of coronaviruses in bats from China. *J Virol*. 2006;80(15):7481–7490.

37. Jahanshahlu L, Rezaei N. Monoclonal antibody as a potential anti-COVID-19. *Biomed Pharmacother*. 2020;129:110337.

38. Amanat F, Krammer F. SARS-CoV-2 vaccines: status report. *Immunity*. 2020;52(4): 583–589.

39. Kamradt-Scott A. WHO's to blame? The World Health Organization and the 2014 Ebola outbreak in West Africa. *Third World Quarterly*. 2016;37(3):401–418.

40. WHO. *Joint External Evaluation Tool: International Health Regulations*; 2016. https://apps.who.int/iris/handle/10665/204368.

41. Green MS, LeDuc J, Cohen D, Franz DR. Confronting the threat of bioterrorism: realities, challenges, and defensive strategies. *Lancet Infect Dis*. 2019;19(1):e2–e13.

Index

Note: Page numbers followed by *f* indicate figures and *t* indicate tables.